Essentials of Cardiovascular Examination

Essentials of Cardiovascular Examination

Sumesh Raj MD
Associate Professor of Internal Medicine
Sree Gokulam Medical College and Research Foundation
Thiruvananthapuram, Kerala, India

Rajan GV BSc MD
Former Professor and Head of Internal Medicine
Government Medical College, Thiruvananthapuram, Kerala, India
Senior Consultant Physician, Cosmopolitan Hospital
Thiruvananthapuram, Kerala, India

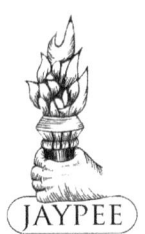

The Health Sciences Publisher
New Delhi | London | Philadelphia | Panama

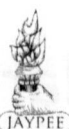 **Jaypee Brothers Medical Publishers (P) Ltd**

Headquarters
Jaypee Brothers Medical Publishers (P) Ltd
4838/24, Ansari Road, Daryaganj
New Delhi 110 002, India
Phone: +91-11-43574357
Fax: +91-11-43574314
Email: jaypee@jaypeebrothers.com

Overseas Offices

J.P. Medical Ltd
83 Victoria Street, London
SW1H 0HW (UK)
Phone: +44-2031708910
Fax: +44 (0)20 3008 6180
Email: info@jpmedpub.com

Jaypee-Highlights Medical Publishers Inc
City of Knowledge, Bld. 237, Clayton
Panama City, Panama
Phone: +1 507-301-0496
Fax: +1 507-301-0499
Email: cservice@jphmedical.com

Jaypee Medical Inc
The Bourse
111 South Independence Mall East
Suite 835, Philadelphia, PA 19106, USA
Phone: +1 267-519-9789
Email: jpmed.us@gmail.com

Jaypee Brothers Medical Publishers (P) Ltd
17/1-B Babar Road, Block-B, Shaymali
Mohammadpur, Dhaka-1207
Bangladesh
Mobile: +08801912003485
Email: jaypeedhaka@gmail.com

Jaypee Brothers Medical Publishers (P) Ltd
Bhotahity, Kathmandu, Nepal
Phone: +977-9741283608
Email: kathmandu@jaypeebrothers.com

Website: www.jaypeebrothers.com
Website: www.jaypeedigital.com

© 2016, Jaypee Brothers Medical Publishers

The views and opinions expressed in this book are solely those of the original contributor(s)/author(s) and do not necessarily represent those of editor(s) of the book.

All rights reserved. No part of this publication may be reproduced, stored or transmitted in any form or by any means, electronic, mechanical, photocopying, recording or otherwise, without the prior permission in writing of the publishers.

All brand names and product names used in this book are trade names, service marks, trademarks or registered trademarks of their respective owners. The publisher is not associated with any product or vendor mentioned in this book.

Medical knowledge and practice change constantly. This book is designed to provide accurate, authoritative information about the subject matter in question. However, readers are advised to check the most current information available on procedures included and check information from the manufacturer of each product to be administered, to verify the recommended dose, formula, method and duration of administration, adverse effects and contraindications. It is the responsibility of the practitioner to take all appropriate safety precautions. Neither the publisher nor the author(s)/editor(s) assume any liability for any injury and/or damage to persons or property arising from or related to use of material in this book.

This book is sold on the understanding that the publisher is not engaged in providing professional medical services. If such advice or services are required, the services of a competent medical professional should be sought.

Every effort has been made where necessary to contact holders of copyright to obtain permission to reproduce copyright material. If any have been inadvertently overlooked, the publisher will be pleased to make the necessary arrangements at the first opportunity.

Inquiries for bulk sales may be solicited at: jaypee@jaypeebrothers.com

Essentials of Cardiovascular Examination

First Edition: **2016**

ISBN 978-93-5250-042-0

Preface

Revolutionary changes are occurring in the field of medical science. New research and clinical experience have broadened our knowledge.

The purpose of this *Essentials of Cardiovascular Examination* is to provide both undergraduate and postgraduate students, interns and practising physicians a solid background in cardiac physical examination.

This book is a humble effort to correct the pitfalls and mistakes that a student commonly makes in undergraduate and postgraduate examinations.

Basic cardiovascular anatomy and physiology are dealt with and correlated with normal and abnormal physical findings elicited at the bedside.

The physical diagnosis is extensively dealt with so as to enable a student for in-depth study and to approach the examination with ease.

All the common cardiovascular diseases and their investigation and treatment updates are also included so as to enable the use of this book as a ready-reckoner reference for practicing physicians.

We acknowledge the untiring effort and help rendered by V Rema Devi, Dr Reshma Sugathan and Sidharth Sumesh in the preparation of this book.

We earnestly appreciate the initiative and effort taken by M/s Jaypee Brothers Medical Publishers (P) Ltd in bringing out this book.

Sumesh Raj
Rajan GV

Contents

Section–A	Approach to the Patient	1–17

Chapter 1   The cardiac history   3
- Chief complaints 3
- Dyspnea 3
- Orthopnea 4
- Paroxysmal nocturnal dyspnea (PND) 4
- Angina pectoris 5
- Palpitation 6
- Syncope 7
- Hemoptysis 8

Chapter 2   General examination in relation to cardiovascular system (CVS)   9
- Head to foot examination 9

Chapter 3   Examination proforma   11
- General examination 11
- Examination of the cardiovascular system 11

Chapter 4   Anatomy of heart and coronary circulation   14
- Embryology of the heart 14
- Anatomy of the heart 14
- Coronary circulation 15
- Venous drainage of the heart 16
- Lymphatic drainage of the heart 16
- Nerve supply of the heart 16

Section–B	Cardiovascular System	19–63

Chapter 5   Arterial pulse   21
- Importance 21
- Method of palpation of the right radial artery 21
- Assessment of arterial pulse 21
- Rhythm 23
- Pulse volume 24

- Pulse character 24
- Pulsus bisferiens 26
- Pulsus alternans 26
- Pulsus bigemini 27
- Pulsus trigemini 27
- Pulsus paradoxus 27
- Reverse pulsus paradoxus 28
- Condition of vessel wall 28
- Examination of peripheral pulses 29
- Radiofemoral delay 29
- Grading of the arterial pulsation 29

Chapter 6 Blood pressure — 30

- Examination of blood pressure 30

Chapter 7 Jugular venous pulse and jugular venous pressure — 32

- Jugular venous pressure 32
- Prerequisites in examination of JVP 32
- JVP as indicator of mean right atrial pressure 32
- Causes of elevated JVP 33
- Causes of fall in JVP 33
- Jugular venous pulse 34

Chapter 8 Inspection of precordium — 37

Chapter 9 Palpation — 39

- Apical impulse 39
- Causes of right ventricular enlargement 41

Chapter 10 Percussion of the heart — 43

Chapter 11 Auscultation — 44

Chapter 12 First heart sound (S_1) — 46

Chapter 13 Second heart sound (S_2) — 48

- Loud S_2 48
- Soft S_2 may be due to soft A_2 or soft P_2 48
- Single S_2 49

- Splitting of S_2 49
- Types of split S_2 50

Chapter 14 Third heart sound (S_3) 51

Chapter 15 Fourth heart sound (S_4) 52

- S_4—atrial contraction sound 52

Chapter 16 Ejection clicks 54

Chapter 17 Heart murmurs 56

- Systolic murmurs 57
- Diastolic murmurs 58
- Continuous murmur 59
- To and fro murmur (biphasic murmur) 61
- Systolic–diastolic murmur 62
- Innocent murmurs 62
- Functional murmurs 62
- Pansystolic murmur (PSM) 63

Section-C Cardiovascular system and related diseases 65–212

Chapter 18 Acute rheumatic fever (ARF) 67

Chapter 19 Infective endocarditis 72

- Acute endocarditis 72
- Prosthetic valve endocarditis (PVE) 73
- Endocarditis occurring among injection drug users 73

Chapter 20 Mitral stenosis (MS) 77

- Juvenile mitral stenosis 78
- Pulmonary edema 79
- Auscultation 79
- Atrial myxoma 82

Chapter 21 Mitral regurgitation (MR) 84

- Mitral regurgitation 84

Chapter 22	**Aortic stenosis (AS)**	88

- Bicuspid aortic valve disease 88
- Silent AS 90

Chapter 23	**Aortic regurgitation (AR)**	93

- Aortic valve involvement 93
- Murmur 95

Chapter 24	**Tricuspid stenosis (TS) and tricuspid regurgitation (TR)**	98

- Tricuspid stenosis (TS) 98
- When to entertain the diagnosis of TS 98
- Tricuspid regurgitation (TR) 99

Chapter 25	**Pulmonary stenosis (PS) and pulmonary regurgitation (PR)**	101

- Pulmonary stenosis (PS) 101
- Pulmonary regurgitation (PR) 102

Chapter 26	**Pulmonary hypertension**	104
Chapter 27	**Mitral valve prolapse (MVP)**	107

- Synonyms 107

Chapter 28	**Atrial septal defect (ASD)**	109
Chapter 29	**Ventricular septal defect (VSD)**	112

- Ventricular septal defect (VSD) 112

Chapter 30	**Patent ductus arteriosus (PDA)**	115
Chapter 31	**Tetralogy of Fallot (TOF)**	117
Chapter 32	**Eisenmenger's syndrome**	121
Chapter 33	**Coarctation of the aorta**	123

- Investigations 124
- Chest radiograph 125
- Doppler echocardiography 125

Chapter 34	**Other congenital heart diseases**	127

- Malpositions of the heart 127

- Total anomalous pulmonary venous connection (TAPVC) 128
- Partial anomalous pulmonary venous connection (PAPVC) 128

Chapter 35 Heart failure (HF) 132

- Classification of cardiac failure 132
- Right and left-sided heart failure and congestive cardiac failure 133
- Forward and backward heart failure 133
- Systolic and diastolic failure 133
- Left ventricular remodeling 134
- Paroxysmal nocturnal dyspnea (PND) 134
- Cheyne-stokes respiration 134
- Drugs for heart failure 138

Chapter 36 Pulmonary thromboembolism (acute cor pulmonale) 140

- Risk factors for deep vein thrombosis 140

Chapter 37 Cor pulmonale (pulmonary heart disease) 144

Chapter 38 Systemic hypertension 148

- Hypertensive crises 148
- Clinical presentation 150

Chapter 39 Ischemic heart disease 154

- Stable angina pectoris 154
- Asymptomatic (silent) ischemia 158

Chapter 40 ST-segment elevation myocardial infarction (STEMI) 159

- Serum cardiac biomarkers 161

Chapter 41 Unstable angina and non-ST-segment elevation myocardial infarction 168

- NSTEMI 168
- Prinzmetal's variant angina 171

Chapter 42	**Arrhythmias**	**172**

- Tachyarrhythmias 172
- Bradyarrhythmias 181

Chapter 43	**Conduction disorders of the heart**	**185**

- Right bundle branch block (RBBB) 185
- Left bundle branch block (LBBB) 186
- Hemiblocks (fascicular blocks) 187

Chapter 44	**Pericardial diseases**	**189**

- Pericarditis 189
- Cardiac tamponade 192
- Chronic constrictive pericarditis 193

Chapter 45	**Myocarditis**	**195**

Chapter 46	**Cardiomyopathy**	**198**

- Types of cardiomyopathy 198
- Dilated cardiomyopathy 198
- Restrictive (obliterative) cardiomyopathy 200
- Hypertrophic obstructive cardiomyopathy (HCM) 201

Chapter 47	**Diseases of the aorta**	**203**

- Aortic aneurysm 203
- Classification aneurysms 203
- Thoracic aortic aneurysms 204
- Abdominal aortic aneurysms 205
- Aortic dissection 206
- Aortitis 206

Chapter 48	**Cardiac manifestations of systemic disease**	**209**

Chapter 49	**Neoplastic diseases of the heart**	**211**

- Primary tumors 211
- Other benign tumors 212

Section-D	**Investigations in Cardiovascular System (CVS)**	**213–229**

Chapter 50	**The electrocardiogram**	**215**

- ECG waveforms and intervals 215

Chapter 51	Noninvasive cardiac imaging		221
	• Echocardiography 221		
	• Radionuclide imaging 222		
	• MRI/CT imaging 222		
Chapter 52	Stress tests		224
Chapter 53	Cardiac catheterization		226
	• Cardiac catheterization 226		

Index   *231*

SECTION A

Approach to the Patient

1. The cardiac history
2. General examination in relation to cardiovascular system (CVS)
3. Examination proforma
4. Anatomy of heart and coronary circulation

Chapter 1

The Cardiac History

Chief Complaints

Symptoms of Cardiovascular Disease
- Chest pain
- Exertional dyspnea
- Orthopnea
- Paroxysmal nocturnal dyspnea (PND)
- Fatigue
- Palpitation
- Syncope
- Hemoptysis.

Dyspnea

Dyspnea is defined as an abnormally uncomfortable awareness of breathing.

New York Heart Association

Classification is for dyspnea, palpitation, fatigue and angina in patients with cardiovascular disease.

Class I — No symptoms with ordinary physical activity
Class II — Slight limitation of physical activity
Class III — Marked limitation of physical activity
Class IV — Symptoms even at rest.

Causes

Cardiac
- Left heart failure
- Congenital heart diseases (shunts and valvular lesions)
- Acquired valvular heart diseases
- Coronary heart disease

- Hypertensive heart disease
- Cardiomyopathies.

Respiratory

a. Bronchial asthma
b. Chronic obstructive lung disease—Chronic bronchitis and emphysema
c. Restrictive lung disease
d. Parenchymal
   - Pneumoconiosis
   - Interstitial lung disease.
e. Extra parenchymal
   - Myasthenia gravis
   - Guillain-Barré syndrome
   - Ankylosing spondylitis
   - Kyphoscoliosis
   - Obesity.
f. Pneumonias
g. Pulmonary neoplasm
h. Pulmonary embolism
i. Laryngeal or tracheal obstruction.
j. Inhalation of toxic gases and fumes

Hematological— Severe anemia.

Miscellaneous—Anxiety and hysterical hyperventilation.

Orthopnea

Dyspnea that develops in recumbent position and is relieved by sitting up.

Mechanism

- When the patient is in a lying down position, the venous return increases. The failing left ventricle is not able to cope with extra volume of blood delivered to it, resulting in increase in pulmonary venous and capillary pressure leading to pulmonary edema.
- Elevated diaphragm in the lying posture decrease the vital capacity of the lung.

Causes

A. Acute left heart failure
B. Extreme degree of congestive cardiac failure (CCF).

Paroxysmal Nocturnal Dyspnea (PND)

- Attacks of dyspnea which occur at night and awaken the patient from sleep.

- It occurs 2–5 hours after the onset of sleep.
- Takes 10–30 minutes for recovery after assuming the upright posture.
- Mechanism of PND is similar to that of orthopnea.
- However, a fall in PaO_2 and a decreased sympathetic support to left ventricular function during sleep also contribute to the development of PND.

Causes
- Ischemic heart disease
- Aortic valve disease
- Hypertension
- Cardiomyopathy
- Atrial fibrillation
- Rarely in mitral disease or atrial tumors.

PND is the Earliest Symptom of Left Heart Failure

Trepopnea

a. Dyspnea occurring in the lateral decubitus position
b. Seen in patients with heart disease.

Platypnea

Platypnea is the dyspnea which occurs only in the upright position.

Causes
- Left atrial thrombus
- Left atrial myxomas
- Pulmonary arteriovenous fistula.

Bendopnea

- Shortness of breath when bending forward such as when putting on their shoes.
- It is a symptom of advanced heart failure.

Angina Pectoris

It is a discomfort in the chest and adjacent area due to myocardial ischemia. It is due to a discrepancy between myocardial oxygen demand and supply.

Canadian Heart Association Grading of Angina

Grade   I   — Angina on severe exertion
Grade II   — Angina on walking uphill
Grade III — Angina on walking on level ground
Grade IV — Angina at rest.

Characteristics of Anginal Pain
- Site—Substernal.
- Nature—Pressing, squeezing, constricting, 'a band across the chest', 'a weight in the center of the chest'.
- The patient cannot pinpoint the site of pain.
- Radiation to both the shoulders, epigastrium, back, neck, jaw and teeth.
- Commonly radiates to the left shoulder and ulnar aspect of the left arm.
- Duration— 5–15 minutes.
- Aggravated by exertion, emotion, after a heavy meal and exposure to cold.
- Relieving factors —Rest and nitrates.

Anginal Equivalent
- Anginal equivalents are symptoms of myocardial ischemia other than angina such as dyspnea, faintness and fatigue.
- They are precipitated by exertion and relieved by rest and nitrates.

Prinzmetal angina
- Typically occurs during rest and may recur in a nightly cyclic pattern
- ST-segment elevation or depression on the electrocardiogram
- Coronary artery spasm has been documented during an attack.

Nocturnal angina
- Angina occurs during sleep at night
- Due to coronary ostial stenosis, as seen in cardiovascular syphilis.

Unstable angina
1. Patients with new onset (< 2 months) angina.
2. Patients with accelerating angina, that is distinctly more frequent, severe and prolonged.
3. Those with angina at rest.

Angina decubitus
Chest pain while lying down.

Palpitation
Palpitation is defined as an unpleasant awareness of rapid heartbeat.

Causes
1. Extrasystoles—Atrial and ventricular
2. Tachyarrhythmias—Atrial and ventricular
3. Endocrine

- Pheochromocytoma
- Thyrotoxicosis
- Hypoglycemia.
4. High output states—Anemia, pyrexia, aortic regurgitation (AR) and PDA
5. Drugs—Atropine, adrenaline, aminophylline and thyroxine
6. Coffee, tea and alcohol
7. Psychogenic — Prolonged anxiety state
8. Idiopathic.

Syncope

Syncope may be defined as a transient loss of consciousness due to inadequate cerebral blood flow.
Secondary to abrupt decrease in cardiac output.
If syncope lasts for—
- 5 seconds, patient experiences dizziness
- 10 seconds, patient may become unconscious
- 15 seconds, patient may throw convulsions.

Causes

Cardiac

- Heart block
- Supraventricular or ventricular tachyarrhythmias
- Aortic stenosis
- Hypertrophic obstructive cardiomyopathy
- Tight mitral stenosis (MS).

Vasovagal syncope

Characteristically occurs in response to fear, sudden emotional stress, anxiety and physical or mental exhaustion.

Orthostatic hypotension

- Produces dizziness on arising or after prolonged standing.
- Due to reduced effective blood volume and autonomic nervous system dysfunction.

Post-tussive (cough) syncope

It occurs with a paroxysm of nonproductive violent coughing, resulting in persistent increase in intrathoracic pressure and decreased venous return to heart and therefore decreased cardiac output.

Micturition syncope

Syncope occurs during or after urination.

Hemoptysis

It occurs in —
- Left ventricular failure (LVF)
- Left atrial failure in mitral stenosis (MS).
Both lead to acute pulmonary edema leading to hemoptysis.

Past History

- Rheumatic fever
- Rheumatic heart disease
- Coronary artery disease (CAD)
- Congenital heart disease
- Hypertension, diabetes and dyslipidemia
- Congenital heart disease
- Prior cardiac surgery
- Thyroid disorder
- Tuberculosis
- Syphilis.

Family History

- Hypertension
- Diabetes
- Coronary artery disease (CAD)
- Hypertrophic obstructive cardiomyopathy (HOCM).

Personal History

Related to diet, smoking and alcoholism.

Treatment History

- History of rheumatic fever prophylaxis
- Digoxin
- Anticoagulant use
- Antihypertensive drugs
- Statins
- Antiplatelet drugs.

Chapter 2

General Examination in Relation to Cardiovascular System (CVS)

- **Stunted growth**—For example, Fallot's tetralogy.
- **Anemia** in infective endocarditis, tetralogy of Fallot (TOF), and prosthetic valve hemolysis.
- **Polycythemia**—Tetralogy of Fallot (TOF).
- **Jaundice**—Infective endocarditis, prosthetic valve hemolysis and cardiac cirrhosis.
- **Clubbing**—Congenital cyanotic heart disease, Eisenmenger's syndrome and infective endocarditis.
- **Differential clubbing**— Posterior descending artery (PDA).
- **Cyanosis**—Congenital cyanotic heart disease and Eisenmenger's syndrome.
- **Edema**—Congestive heart failure (CCF) and right heart failure.

Head to Foot Examination

Look for—
- Peripheral signs of aortic regurgitation (AR)
- Signs of rheumatic fever—
  - Migrating polyarthritis
  - Erythema marginatum
  - Subcutaneous nodules
  - Sydenham's chorea.

Marfanoid Features

- Upper segment/lower segment inequality
- Arachnodactyly
- High arched palate
- Wrist sign
- Thumb sign.

Signs of Infective Endocarditis
- Anemia and jaundice
- Clubbing and splinter hemorrhages
- Osler's nodes
- Janeway lesions
- Arthritis.

Embolic complications of infective endocarditis
- Osler's node — Painful, purple and pea-shaped nodule
- Janeway lesion — Painless
- Splinter hemorrhage.

Markers of Coronary Heart Disease
- Arcus senilis
- Xanthelasma and xanthomas
- Earlobe creases — Diagonal
- Nicotine stains on fingers and teeth
- Obesity
- Thyroid enlargement.

Also look for—
- Hypertelorism
- Low set ears
- High arched palate
- Webbed neck
- Syndactyly, polydactyly and arachnodactyly
- Cubitus valgus
- Absent radius
- Pectus excavatum and carinatum
- Kyphoscoliosis
- Dwarfism
- Gigantism.

Look for Down, Turner's and Klinefelter's syndromes.
- Fundus—Look for
    a. Infective endocarditis—Roth's spot
    b. Hypertensive retinopathy
    c. Papilledema in malignant hypertension
    d. Retinal artery pulsations in AR (Becker's sign).

Chapter 3

Examination Proforma

General Examination

- Built and nourishment
- Pallor
- Icterus
- Cyanosis
- Clubbing
- Edema
- Lymphadenopathy.

Head to Foot Examination

Vital signs
- Pulse
- Blood pressure
- Respiratory rate
- Temperature.

Examination of the Cardiovascular System

Examination of the Arterial Pulse

Examination of the right radial artery

Look for—
1. Rate
2. Rhythm
3. Volume
4. Character
5. Radiofemoral delay
6. Condition of vessel wall.

Examination of Blood Pressure

- In both upper limbs.
- Measure lower limb blood pressure.
- Look for orthostatic hypotension.
- Note the blood pressure in supine position. Ask the patient to stand upright for 3 minutes. Note the blood pressure. If the fall in systolic blood pressure is >20 mmHg or diastolic is >10 mmHg with or without symptoms, it is indicative of orthostatic hypotension.

Blood pressure in atrial fibrillation

An average of 2–3 readings are taken.

Examination of Jugular Venous Pressure, Jugular Venous Pulse and Hepatojugular Reflux

Inspection

- Shape of precordium
- Position of the apex
- Dilated veins
- Visible pulsations.

Palpation

1. Palpation of the apical impulse
2. Left parasternal heave
3. Epigastric pulsations
4. Palpation of pulmonary arterial pulsation
5. Other palpable events
   a. Prominent aortic pulsations (as in aortic aneurysm).
   b. Pulsations of LV aneurysm or dyskinetic segment may be felt above and medial to the apex.
6. Thrills.

Percussion

Percussion of the right, left border and base of the heart—The left border of the heart corresponds to the apex beat, the right border to the right sternal border and base of heart in 2nd space.

Percussion of dullness in the 2nd space—Normally does not extent beyond 2.5 cm on either side of the sternum.

Auscultation
- For heart sounds, murmurs and ejection click
- Pulse deficit
- Auscultation over the carotids
- Auscultation over the back and supraclavicular areas.

Chapter 4

Anatomy of Heart and Coronary Circulation

Embryology of the Heart

- The heart is the first organ to form during embryogenesis.
- Early cardiac precursors form 2 bilateral heart tubes, each composed of a single cell layer of endocardium surrounded by a single layer of myocardial precursors (Fig. 4.1).
- Subsequently, a single midline heart tube is formed by the medial migration and midline fusion of these bilateral structures.
- The caudal, inflow region of the heart tube and represents the atrial structures, whereas the rostral, outflow portion of the tube forms the truncus arteriosus, which divides to produce the aorta and the proximal pulmonary artery.
- Between these extremes lie the structural precursors of the ventricles.

Anatomy of the Heart

The heart is located just behind and slightly left of the sternum. The heart has four chambers (Fig. 4.2):
- The right atrium receives blood from the superior and inferior vena cavae and pumps it to the right ventricle.

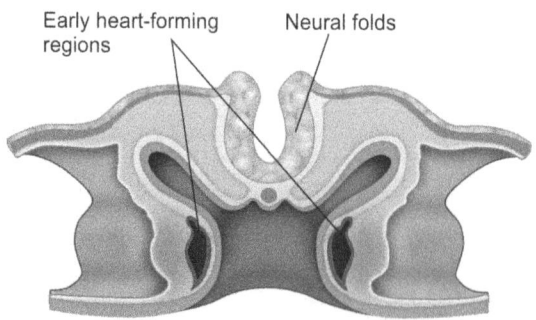

Fig. 4.1: Formation of heart tubes

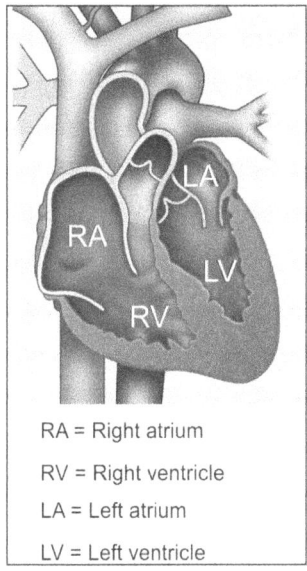

RA = Right atrium
RV = Right ventricle
LA = Left atrium
LV = Left ventricle

Fig. 4.2: Cross section of heart

- The right ventricle receives blood from the right atrium and pumps blood through the pulmonary artery to the lungs.
- The left atrium receives oxygenated blood from the lungs through the 4 pulmonary veins and pumps it to the left ventricle.
- The left ventricle pumps oxygen-rich blood to the rest of the body through the aorta.

The heart is surrounded by pericardium which has a parietal and visceral layer.

Coronary Circulation

- The left coronary artery originates from the left aortic sinus, while the right coronary artery originates from the right aortic sinus.
- The left coronary artery divides into the left anterior descending artery and circumflex artery.
- It supplies the lateral and anterior walls of the left ventricle, and the anterior two-thirds of the interventricular septum.
- Left anterior descending (LAD) coronary artery travels down the anterior interventricular groove.
- The LAD gives off 2 types of branches: Septals and diagonals.
- LAD is also known as widow's artery.
- Right coronary artery traverses the atrioventricular groove or the coronary sulcus.

- It branches into the posterior descending artery and the right marginal artery.
- At the origin of the right coronary artery (RCA) is the conus artery.
- The RCA supplies the right ventricle, the posterior wall of the left ventricle and posterior-third of the septum.
- The posterior discending artery (PDA) supplies the inferior wall, ventricular septum and the posteromedial papillary muscle.
- The RCA also supplies the SA nodal artery in 60% of patients. The other 40% of the time, the SA nodal artery is supplied by the left circumflex artery. The atrioventricular nodal branch most frequently arises as a distal branch from the right coronary artery.

Coronary Artery Dominance

The artery that supplies the PDA determines the coronary dominance.
- If the PDA is supplied by the RCA, then the coronary circulation can be classified as "right-dominant".
- If the PDA is supplied by the circumflex artery (CX), a branch of the left artery, then the coronary circulation can be classified as "left-dominant".
- If the PDA is supplied by both the RCA and the circumflex artery, then the coronary circulation can be classified as "co-dominant".
Approximately 70% of the general population are right-dominant.

Venous Drainage of the Heart

- The venous system follows the coronary arteries and drains into the coronary sinus.
- The coronary sinus runs transversely in the left atrioventricular groove on the posterior side of the heart. It is the distal portion of the great cardiac vein feeding into the right atrium.
- The coronary sinus receives blood mainly from the small, middle, great and oblique cardiac veins.
- The coronary sinus drains into the right atrium.

Lymphatic Drainage of the Heart

An extensive lymphatic system drains into vessels that travel with the coronary vessels and then into the thoracic duct.

Nerve Supply of the Heart

The heart is innervated by parasympathetic and sympathetic fibers.

Sympathetic Nervous System

Sympathetic nerves from the cervical sympathetic chain travel along arteries and nerves and are found in the adventitia of blood vessels. Sympathetic efferent nerves are present throughout the atria, ventricles (including the conduction system), and myocytes in the heart and also the sinoatrial (SA) and atrioventricular (AV) nodes.

Parasympathetic Nervous System

Parasympathetic preganglionic fibers reach the heart through the vagus nerve.

The parasympathetic nervous system mainly innervates the SA and AV nodes in the heart. Atrial muscle is also innervated by vagal efferents.

SECTION B

Cardiovascular System

5. Arterial pulse
6. Blood pressure
7. Jugular venous pulse and jugular venous pressure
8. Inspection of precordium
9. Palpation
10. Percussion of the heart
11. Auscultation
12. First heart sound (S_1)
13. Second heart sound (S_2)
14. Third heart sound (S_3)
15. Fourth heart sound (S_4)
16. Ejection clicks
17. Heart murmurs

Chapter 5

Arterial Pulse

Definition

Arterial pulse is a waveform that is felt by the finger, produced by cardiac systole; which traverses the arterial tree in a peripheral direction.

Importance

It gives information about
1. Condition of the vessel wall
2. Rough estimate of systolic blood pressure
3. State of the heart and circulation
4. Diagnosis of arrhythmias
5. Diagnosis of pathological entities like AR and LVF.

It has been called the mirror or index of the heart.

Method of Palpation of the Right Radial Artery

Position of the Patient

Patient should be in supine position, arms slightly flexed at the elbow, forearm semipronated, wrist slightly flexed, support the patient's hand with examiner's right hand and palpate radial artery against the head of radius with 3 fingers of the left hand and count for 1 minute.

Assessment of Arterial Pulse

Arterial pulse is examined in the following way
1. Rate
2. Rhythm
3. Volume
4. Character
5. Tension
6. Condition of the vessel wall
7. Whether all peripheral pulses felt equally and bilaterally

8. Radiofemoral delay
   - Radial pulse is felt to assess rate and rhythm
   - Carotid pulse is felt to assess volume and character
   - Brachial pulse is felt to record blood pressure.

Table 5.1: Timing of pulse wave with cardiac systole

Artery	Time at which pulse wave arrives after cardiac systole
Carotid	30 milliseconds
Brachial	60 milliseconds
Femoral	75 milliseconds
Radial	80 milliseconds

Pulse Rate

- Pulse rate should be counted for one full minute by palpating the radial artery.
- Normal pulse rate is 60–100/minute.
- Sinus bradycardia—Pulse rate < 60/minute.
- Sinus tachycardia—Pulse rate > 100/minute.

Causes of Sinus Bradycardia

Physiological

- Athletes
- During sleep.

Pathological

- Severe hypoxia
- Hypothermia
- Sick sinus syndrome
- Obstructive jaundice
- Myxedema
- Acute inferior wall myocardial infarction
- Raised intraocular pressure
- Raised intracranial tension
- Heart block
- Drugs (betablockers, verapamil, diltiazem and digoxin).

Causes of Sinus Tachycardia

Physiological

- Infants
- Children

- Emotion
- Exertion
- Anxiety.

Pathological

1. Tachyarrhythmias—Supraventricular and ventricular.
2. High output states—Anemia, pyrexia, beriberi, thyrotoxicosis, pheochromocytoma and acute anterior wall myocardial infarction.
3. Cardiac failure and cardiogenic shock.
4. Hypovolemia, hypotension and atrial fibrillation.
5. Drugs (atropine, nifedipine, β-agonists—Salbutamol, L-thyroxine, catecholamines, nicotine and caffeine).

Pulse Deficit

It is the difference between the heart rate and the pulse rate when counted simultaneously for one full minute.

How to look for

For this simultaneously count the heart rate, which is examined by another examiner and pulse rate (which is examined by the first examiner).

Causes

Atrial fibrillation (AF) and ventricular premature beats (VPC).

Table 5.2: Differences between VPCs and AF

Features	VPCs	AF
Pulse deficit	Less than 10/minute	More than 10/minute
A wave in JVP	Present	Absent
On exertion	Decreases or disappears	Persists or increases
Rhythm	Short pause between normal beat and VPC	Pauses are variable

Rhythm

Rhythm is assessed by palpating the radial artery.

Sinus Arrhythmia

1. Common in childhood, because of overaction of vagus nerve, it is sometimes referred to as juvenile irregularity of the heart.
2. Rhythm may be regular or irregular.

Regularly Irregular Rhythm

Seen in—

1. Atrial tachyarrhythmias— Paroxysmal atrial tachycardia (PAT) and atrial flutter with fixed atrioventricular (AV) block.
2. Ventricular bigemini and trigemini.

Irregularly Irregular Rhythm

Seen in—
1. Atrial or ventricular ectopics
2. Atrial fibrillation
3. PAT and atrial flutter with varying AV block.

Pulse Volume

Examined by the trisection method. Three varying degree of pressure is applied to the pulse with finger while concentrating on separate phases of the pulse wave: Upstroke, systolic peak and diastolic slope.

Pulse volume is best assessed by palpating the carotid artery. However the pulse pressure, the difference between systolic and diastolic blood pressure gives accurate measure of pulse volume. When pulse pressure is between 30 and 60 mmHg, pulse volume is normal. When pulse pressure is less than 30 mmHg, it is a small volume pulse. When pulse pressure is greater than 60 mmHg, it is a large volume pulse.

Pulse volume depends on stroke volume and arterial compliance.

Pulse Character

Pulse character is best assessed in the carotid arteries.

Anacrotic Pulse

(Pulsus Parvus et. Tardus) (Fig. 5.1).

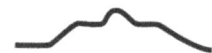

Fig. 5.1: Anacrotic pulse

A low amplitude pulse (Parvus) with a slow rising and late peak. Seen in severe aortic stenosis (AS).

Dicrotic Pulse (Fig. 5.2)

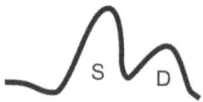

Fig. 5.2: Dicrotic pulse

One peak in systole, another in diastole.

Causes
1. LVF
2. Enteric fever
3. Dehydration
4. Dilated cardiomyopathy
5. Cardiac tamponade.

Hypokinetic Pulse (Fig. 5.3)

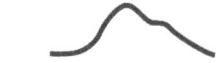

Fig. 5.3: Hypokinetic pulse

1. Low volume pulse.
2. Small weak pulse (small volume and narrow pulse).

Causes

Cardiac failure, shock, mitral stenosis and aortic stenosis.

Hyperkinetic Pulse (Fig. 5.4)

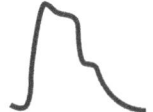

Fig. 5.4: Hyperkinetic pulse

High volume pulse (pulsus magnus) with a rapid rise, large volume and wide pulse pressure.
Seen in—
1. In high output state—Anemia, pyrexia and beriberi.
2. Mitral regurgitation (MR) and ventricular septal defect (VSD).

Collapsing Pulse (Fig. 5.5)
1. It is a large volume pulse. There is a rapid upstroke and rapid downstroke.
2. Systolic pressure is high and diastolic pressure is low.

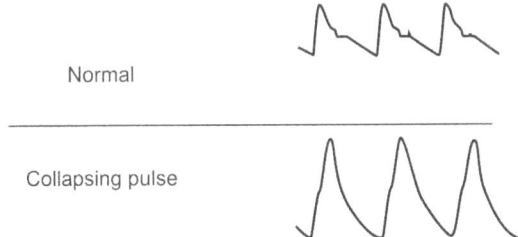

Fig. 5.5: Normal pulse and collapsing pulse

Causes

It occurs in AR, PDA, RSOV and AV fistula.

How to look for

Patient is made to lie in supine position, feel for the right radial artery with distal aspect of the examiner's palm. Elevate the hand vertically to feel for a thud or collapse.

Mechanism

The rapid upstroke is because of an increased stroke volume. The rapid downstroke is because of diastolic run off into the ventricle and decreased peripheral resistance leading to rapid run off to the periphery.

Described by Corrigan, water hammer is a 19th century toy, sealed-glass tube containing water and vacuum. On inversion water would suddenly drop through vacuum imparting a palpable shock.

Thready Pulse

Small amplitude pulse in peripheral circulatory failure and shock.

Jerky Pulse

It is seen in hypertrophic obstructive cardiomyopathy (HOCM).

Pseudocollapsing Pulse

- It is a normal volume collapsing pulse
- Seen in mitral regurgitation.

Pulsus Bisferiens (Fig. 5.6)

Double peak in systole.

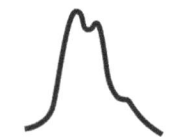

Fig. 5.6: Pulsus bisferiens

Causes

- Severe AR
- AS with AR
- HOCM.

Pulsus Alternans (Fig. 5.7)

Alternating small and large volume pulse in regular rhythm. It is best appreciated by palpating radial or femoral pulses.

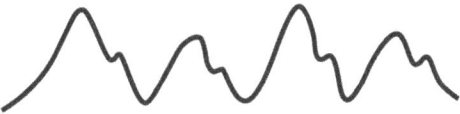

Fig. 5.7: Pulsus alternans

Causes

1. Severe LVF
2. Following VPC.
- It may occur following paroxysmal tachycardia.
- Pulses alternans may be associated with S_3 and electrical alternans: Alternate small and large ECG complexes (in 10% cases).

How to Look for

Patient lies in supine position and femoral or radial artery is palpated with fingers using light pressure and breath held in midexpiration.

Patient lies in supine position. Cuff inflated 15 mmHg suprasystolic. Deflate slowly until first beats are heard. Hold at that point in normal respiration. Sounds produced by the stronger beats alone are heard. Note the BP. Slowly deflate till sounds are heard as though they are doubled (doubling of Korotkoff sounds). Note the BP difference. If >20 mmHg it can be appreciated in the pulse.

Pulsus Bigemini (Fig. 5.8)

A pulse wave with a normal beat followed by a premature beat and a compensatory pause occurring is rapid succession resulting in alteration of the strength of the pulse. In pulses alternans compensatory pause is absent. Pulses bigeminus is a sign of digitalis toxicity.

Pulsus Trigemini

A pulse wave with 2 normal beats followed by a premature beat.

Pulsus Paradoxus

It is an exaggerated reduction of the strength of arterial pulse during normal inspiration or an exaggerated inspiratory fall in systolic pressure of more than 10 mmHg during quiet breathing.

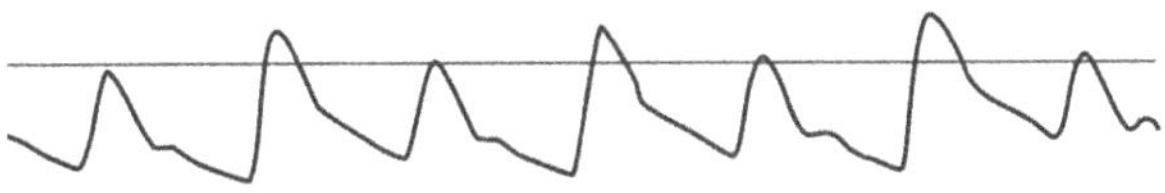

Fig. 5.8: Pulsus bigemini

Causes

1. Cardiac tamponade
2. Constrictive pericarditis
3. Airway obstruction—Acute severe asthma and COPD
4. SVC obstruction.

How to Look for

Patient lies in the supine position. Cuff is inflated 15 mmHg above the systolic blood pressure. Deflate slowly until first beats are heard. Hold at that point in normal respiration. Sounds will be heard only during expiration. Note the blood pressure. Slowly deflate till the sounds are heard during both inspiration and expiration. Note the blood pressure. The difference between the two more than 10 mmHg indicates pulsus paradoxus. If the blood pressure difference is >20 mmHg it can be felt in the pulse.

Reverse Pulsus Paradoxus

It is an inspiratory rise in arterial pressure.

Causes

- HOCM
- Intermittent positive pressure ventilation
- Atrioventricular dissociation.

Intermittent Pulse

Intermittent dropping out of beats at the pulse.

Tension of the Pulse

- Corresponds to diastolic blood pressure.
- In low tension pulse (pulsus mollis)—Vessel is soft and impalpable between beats.
- In high tension pulse (pulsus durus)—Vessel is cord-like.

Condition of Vessel Wall

How to Look for

Patient lied supine. Palpate the radial artery with 3 fingers. Compress the radial artery with proximal finger, empty the vessel with the distal finger and roll the vessel over the head of the radius to feel the vessel wall.

In long standing hypertension, arteriosclerotic change produces a rigid-pipe stem artery.

Examination of Peripheral Pulses

Method of Palpation

Always compare both sides for any differences.
- **Carotid arteries**: Patient in supine position: Gently palpate the carotid artery with 3 fingers of the right hand or with the left thumb at the level of the thyroid cartilage against the transverse process of the cervical vertebrae. Both the carotids should not be palpated simultaneously.
- **Femoral artery**: With patient lying supine, feel the artery with the thumb or fingers just below the midpoint between anterior-superior iliac crest and pubic tubercle, against the neck of the femur.
- **Popliteal artery**: Patient lies in supine position. Keep the knee flexed at 120°. Feel for the popliteal artery in medial part of popliteal fossa with the fingertips of both hands, with the thumb resting on the patient's patella.
- **Posterior tibial artery**: Palpated 1 cm behind the medial malleolus with foot relaxed between plantar and dorsiflexion.
- **Dorsalis pedis artery**: Palpate against the tarsal bones. Left dorsalis pedis is examined with fingers of right hand with examiner on the right side and vice versa.

Radiofemoral Delay

Delay in the femoral compared with the radial pulse is found in coarctation of the aorta.

Grading of the Arterial Pulsation

Grade 0	—Absent
Grade 1+	—Feeble/low
Grade 2+	—Normal
Grade 3+	—High/bounding pulse.

Chapter 6

Blood Pressure

Examination of Blood Pressure

Patient should be resting (relaxed) 5 minutes in a chair or in supine position.

All Clothing should be Removed from the Arm

Avoid bladder distension, caffeine, exercise, eating and smoking half an hour before the examination.

Once the cuff is placed on the arm; the cuff on the arm, the sphygmomanometer and the examiner's eye should be at the same level. Cuff should be applied closely to the upper arm with the lower border more than 2.5 cm from the cubital fossa. Cuff width should be 40% of arm circumference and length 80% of the arm circumference. Ratio of width to length is 1:2.

- Standard size of cuff for upper limb is: 12 × 24 cm
- For thigh it is: 18 × 36 cm.

Patient is relaxed in a chair or supine position and arm supported at the level of the heart. Tubing of the cuff should be along the brachial artery.

The cuff is inflated and simultaneously palpate the radial pulse. Inflate the cuff so that the radial pulse is no longer felt. Increase the pressure 30 mmHg more. Place the diaphragm of stethoscope lightly over the brachial artery (excess pressure can decrease the diastolic blood pressure). Deflate slowly at 2-3 mm/second or per heartbeat, until the Korotkoff sounds are heard. Phase I or clear tapping is the systolic blood pressure. Phase V or disappearance of the sound is true diastolic blood pressure (except in AR where the difference in phase IV and V is >10 mmHg, then phase IV is taken as the diastolic blood pressure). If sounds are inaudible it is accentuated by opening and closing the fist (to dilate the blood vessels).

Difference in blood pressure of the right and left upper limbs of >10 mmHg is significant (blood pressure is higher in the dominant limb due to increased muscle mass).

- *Lower limb blood pressure*: It can be examined in the midthigh or calf.
- **Midthigh**: Patient should lie in the prone position. Hold the knee slightly flexed to relax the muscles around the popliteal fossa. Cuff should be rolled diagonally around the thigh to keep the edges snugged against the skin. Palpate the popliteal artery and then auscultate it.
- **Calf**: Place the cuff in midcalf, diagonally and palpate the posterior tibial and auscultate it.

Pulsus Paradoxus

Patient lies in the supine position. Cuff is inflated 15 mmHg above the apparent highest systolic blood pressure. Deflate slowly until first beats are heard. Hold at that point in normal respiration. Sounds will be heard only during expiration. Note the blood pressure. Slowly deflate till the sounds are heard during both inspiration and expiration. Note the blood pressure. The difference between the two more than 10 mmHg indicates pulsus paradoxus. If the blood pressure difference is >20 mmHg it can be felt in the pulse.

Pulsus Alternans

Patient lies in supine position. Cuff inflated 15 mmHg suprasystolic. Deflate slowly until first beats are heard. Hold at that point in normal respiration. Sounds produced by the stronger beats alone are heard. Note the blood pressure. Slowly deflate till sounds are heard as though they are doubled (doubling of Korotkoff sounds). Note the blood pressure difference. If >20 mmHg it can be appreciated in the pulse.

Orthostatic Hypotension

Note the blood pressure in supine position. Ask the patient to stand upright for 3 minutes. Note the blood pressure. If the fall systolic blood pressure is >20 mmHg or diastolic or >10 mmHg with or without symptoms, it is indicative of orthostatic hypotension.

Blood Pressure in Atrial Fibrillation

An average of 2–3 readings are taken.

Chapter 7

Jugular Venous Pulse and Jugular Venous Pressure

Jugular Venous Pressure (Fig. 7.1)

- Jugular venous pressure (JVP) is height of the vertical column of blood in the right internal jugular vein measured from the sternal angle of Louis.
- When measured with the patient reclining at 45° is normally about 4–5 cm.
- The right internal jugular vein is selected because it is larger, straighter and has no valves. It is situated between two heads of sternomastoid.

Prerequisites in Examination of JVP

- Patient lies comfortably in an examination table.
- Clothing removed from neck and upper thorax.
- Head should rest on a pillow, but at no sharp angulation with trunk.
- Daylight is preferred. But tangential light across the neck can silhouette the neck veins to great advantage.
- Examined at 45° on examination table.
- But if the pressure is high, a higher inclination of 60° or 90° is required to obtain the visible pulsation.

JVP as Indicator of Mean Right Atrial Pressure

- The overall height of the pulsating column is an indicator of mean right atrial pressure.
- In most individuals, the center of the right atrium is approximately 5 cm from the sternal angle of Louis.

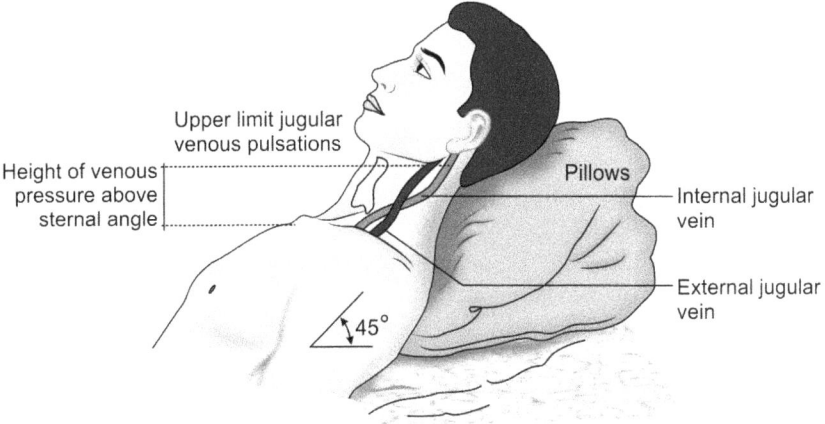

Fig. 7.1: Position for examination of JVP

- Thus, the vertical height of the column of blood in the neck can be estimated from the sterna angle, to which 5 cm is added to obtain an estimate of mean right atrial pressure in centimeters of blood.
- Normal values are less than 8 cm of blood or less than 6 mmHg.

Causes of Elevated JVP

Cardiac
- Cardiac failure
- Tricuspid stenosis
- Tricuspid regurgitation
- Constrictive pericarditis
- Cardiac tamponade.

Pulmonary
Chronic obstructive pulmonary disease (COPD)/cor pulmonale.

Abdominal
- Ascites
- Pregnancy.

Iatrogenic—Excess IV Fluids
- Most common cause of raised JVP is CCF
- Elevated nonpulsatile JVP is seen in SVC obstruction.

Causes of Fall in JVP

- Hypovolemia

- Shock
- Addison's disease.

Jugular Venous Pulse

- The venous pulse has three positive waves, 'a', 'c' and 'v', and two negative waves or descents, 'x' and 'y' (Fig. 7.2).
- A wave is due to atrial contraction (Table 7.1).
- This is followed by the 'x' descent, which is interrupted by a small 'c' wave which is rarely visible on inspection of the neck veins.
- The 'c' wave coincides with the onset of ventricular systole and results from tricuspid valve closure.
- The 'v' wave indicates a passive rise in pressure as venous return continues while the tricuspid valve is closed.
- The 'y' descent—When the tricuspid valve opens, blood enters the right ventricle rapidly and there is consequently a lowering of the right atrial pressure.

Table 7.1: Cardiac events in relation to waves in JVP

Waves in JVP	Cardiac event
'a' wave (atrial wave)	Right atrial contraction
'c' wave (closure wave)	Carotid artery impact
Tricuspid valve ascends	
'x' descent	Right atrial relaxation
Tricuspid valve descends	
'v' wave (ventricular wave)	Venous filling into atrium
'y' descent	Tricuspid valve opens

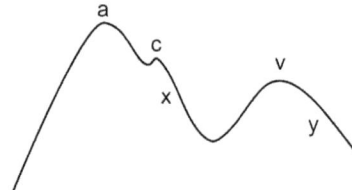

Fig. 7.2: Waves in JVP

Table 7.2: Differentiating features between JVP and carotid pulse

JVP (Pulse)	Carotid pulse
Varies with posture	Does not change

Contd...

Contd...

JVP (Pulse)	Carotid pulse
Changes with respiration	Does not change
Multiple upstroke	Single upstroke
Predominant inward movement	Predominant outward movement
Obliterable	Nonobliterable
Better visible	Better palpable
Two peaks per heartbeat	One peak per heartbeat
Seen in the triangle formed by the two heads of the sternomastoid and the clavicle	Seen internal to the sternomastoid

Abnormalities of JVP

'a' wave
- **Absent**—Atrial fibrillation.
- Prominent 'a' waves
  - Pulmonary stenosis
  - Pulmonary hypertension
  - Tricuspid atresia or stenosis.
- 'a' wave occurs before the carotids.
- 'v' wave occurs with or just after the carotids.

Cannon Waves (Giant 'a' Waves Seen)

- Regular junctional rhythm
- Irregular multiple ectopics
- Complete heart block
  - 'v' wave prominent in tricuspid regurgitation.
  - 'x' descent prominent in constrictive pericarditis.
  - 'y' descent slow in tricuspid stenosis.
  - **Rapid 'y' descent**—Friedreich's sign in constrictive pericarditis and tricuspid regurgitation (TR).
  - **Kussmaul's sign** is an inspiratory increase in JVP.

Causes of Kussmaul's Sign

- Constrictive pericarditis
- Restrictive cardiomyopathy
- Right ventricle infarct
- Right ventricle failure.

Hepatojugular Reflux

- Firm compression is given in the mid abdomen for 30 seconds.

- In normal individuals the JVP rises transiently by less than 3 cm and falls down even when pressure is continued, whereas in patients with right heart failure, the JVP remains elevated.
- It is positive in right heart failure and tricuspid regurgitation.
- It is negative in Budd-Chiari syndrome.

Chapter 8

Inspection of Precordium

Precordium is the anterior aspect of chest overlying the heart.

Table 8.1: Chest wall defects

Sternum	Pectus excavatum (Cobbler's chest)
	Pectus carinatum (Pigeon chest)
Costal cartilages	Costochondritis
Spine	Kyphosis
	Scoliosis
	Ankylosing spondylitis
	Straight back syndrome

Visible Pulsations

Aortic pulsation
- Dilatation of ascending aorta
- Aortic aneurysm
- Aortic regurgitation (AR).

Pulmonary artery pulsation
- Pulmonary artery dilatation
- High output states
- Pulmonary hypertension.

Suprasternal pulsation
- AR
- Aortic arch aneurysm
- Thyrotoxicosis
- Coarctation of aorta.

Left parasternal pulsation
Right ventricular hypertrophy.

Apical pulsation

Left ventricular or right ventricular enlargement.

Inter and infrascapular pulsations

Coarctation of aorta (Suzman's sign).

Epigastric pulsation

- Aortic aneurysm (expansile pulsation)
- Right ventricular hypertrophy.

Hepatic pulsation

- Tricuspid stenosis
- Tricuspid regurgitation
- AR.

Chapter 9

Palpation

- The fingertips are used to feel pulsations
- The base of fingers for thrills
- Hand base for heaves
- Ideal position is supine.

Apical Impulse

- Apical impulse is the lowermost and outermost point of the chest wall where a definite cardiac impulse is felt.
- Normal apical impulse is produced by left ventricle and the left ventricular portion of the interventricular septum.
- Normal site of the apical impulse is about 1 cm medial to midclavicular line at the left 5th intercostal space in adults.
- Normal displacement is 1 cm laterally in left lateral decubitus position.
- Normal apical impulse is confined to one intercostals space and has an area of 2.5 cm².
- Normal duration of thrust of apical impulse is less than 1/3rd of systole.
- When the apical impulse is not localizable on the left side, palpate the right hemithorax for dextrocardia.

Abnormalities of Apical Impulse

Absent apical impulse

- Behind the rib or sternum
- Dextrocardia
- Emphysema
- Obesity
- Thick chest wall.

Tapping apical impulse

- In mitral stenosis
- Palpable S_1.

Hypodynamic apical impulse (felt with decreased thrust)

Seen in—
- Acute myocardial infarction
- Obesity
- Pleural effusion
- Pericardial effusion
- Constrictive pericarditis
- COPD
- Pneumothorax.

Hyperdynamic apical impulse
- There is an increase in amplitude without an increase in duration
- Seen in AR and MR.

Heaving apical impulse
- It is one in which there is increase in both amplitude and duration
- Seen in aortic stenosis (AS).

Diffuse apical impulse

Seen in—
- Left ventricular aneurysm
- Left ventricular dysfunction.

Double apical impulse
- HOCM
- Left ventricular aneurysm
- AS with AR
- Left bundle branch block.

Triple or quadruple apical impulse
- HOCM.

Retractile apical impulse
- Constrictive pericarditis
- Severe TR.

Heaving apical impulse
- Duration— > 2/3rd of systole.
- Occupies one intercostal space.
- Causes— Left ventricular (LV) pressure overload, e.g. aortic stenosis (AS), HTN and coarctation of aorta.

Hyperdynamic apical impulse
- Duration — < 2/3rd of systole.
- Occupies more than one intercostal space.
- Seen in conditiond of LV volume overload like AR, MR, VSD, PDA and high output states.

Left parasternal impulse

Parasternal impulse is the anterior movement of lower-left parasternal area.

Grading of parasternal impulse
- Grade I—Visible
- Grade II—Palpable but obliterable
- Grade III—Palpable but not obliterable.

Left parasternal heave can be seen in—
- Right ventricular hypertrophy
- Gross left atrial enlargement.

Causes of Right Ventricular Enlargement

ASD, VSD, PS and PAH.

Left Atrial Enlargement
- Left atrial enlargement is seen in mitral stenosis and mitral regurgitation.
- Aneurysmal dilatation of LA (giant LA) is seen in severe mitral regurgitation.

Shocks
- Shocks are palpable equivalents of heart sounds
- Palpable A_2 in aortic area in systemic hypertension
- Palpable P_2 in pulmonary area in pulmonary hypertension
- Palpable S_1 in apical area in mitral stenosis.

Thrills
- Thrills are palpable vibrations in time with cardiac cycle.
- They are palpable equivalents of heart murmurs.
- The presence of a thrill indicates that the murmur is most of the time organic.
- As a general rule, apical thrills are diastolic and basal thrills are systolic.
- Apical thrill may be systolic (as in severe MR) and basal thrills may be diastolic (as in acute severe AR).

- Carotid thrill (carotid shudder)—In aortic stenosis, systolic thrill is palpated over the carotids.
- Systolic thrill in aortic area in aortic stenosis.
- Diastolic thrill in aortic area in AR.
- Systolic thrill in pulmonary area in pulmonary stenosis, ASD, ventricular septal defect and patent ductus arteriosus.
- Continuous thrill in pulmonary area in patent ductus arteriosus and rupture of sinus of Valsalva.
- Diastolic thrill in apex in mitral stenosis.
- Systolic thrill in apex in mitral regurgitation and aortic stenosis.

Chapter 10
Percussion of the Heart

Percussion of
1. Right border—It corresponds to right sternal border
2. Left border—It corresponds to the apex
3. Base of the heart—It corresponds to the 2nd space
4. Helpful for finding out the position and enlargement of heart as in—
   - Dextrocardia
   - Pericardial effusion
   - Dilated cardiomyopathy.

Percussion of Second Space Dullness
- Normally dullness extends upto 2.5 cm on either side of the sternum.
- It is useful in detecting aortic dilatation as in aneurysm of aorta and pulmonary artery dilatation as in pulmonary hypertension or idiopathic pulmonary artery dilatation.

Chapter 11

Auscultation

Features of an Ideal Stethoscope

- Tube of length — 25 cm
- Diaphragm diameter — 4 cm
- Bell diameter — 2.5 cm

Bell of Stethoscope

It is used to auscultate—
- Low-pitched sounds and murmurs
- Third heart sound
- Fourth heart sound
- Mid-diastolic murmurs.

Diaphragm of Stethoscope

It is used to auscultate—
- High-pitched sounds and murmurs
- First heart sound
- Second heart sound
- Clicks
- Opening snaps
- Tumor plops
- Pericardial rubs and knocks
- Systolic murmurs
- Early diastolic murmurs.

Areas of Auscultation (Fig.11.1)

- Mitral area corresponds to cardiac apex.
- Tricuspid area corresponds to the lower-left parasternal area.
- Aortic area corresponds to the 2nd right intercostals space close to the sternum.

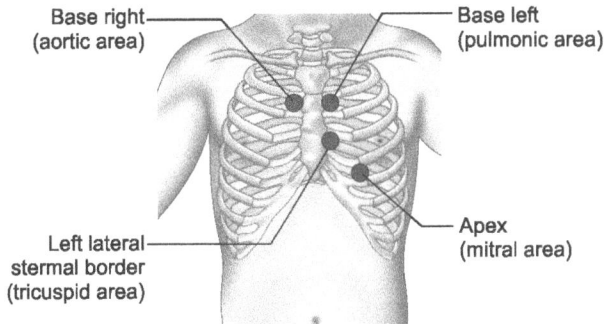

Fig. 11.1: Areas of auscultation

- Pulmonary area corresponds to the 2nd left intercostal space close to the sternum.
- Erb's area (second aortic area) corresponds to 3rd left intercostal space close to the sternum.
- Gibson's area corresponds to left first intercostals space close to sternum. PDA murmur is best heard here (Gibson's murmur).

The heart is auscultated for—
1. Heart sounds
2. Presence of murmurs
3. Presence of added sounds (S_3, S_4, OS, pericardial rub, diastolic knock, tumor plop and prosthetic valve sounds).

Chapter 12

First Heart Sound (S_1)

The first heart sound (S_1) is produced by closure of the mitral (M_1) and tricuspid valves (T_1).

It corresponds to the end of diastole and beginning of ventricular systole and precedes the upstroke of carotid pulsation. Refer to the audio example below.

M_1 is best heard over the apex of the heart, and T_1 is best heard over the fourth ICS at the left sternal border.

Conditions associated with a loud S_1 include the followings:
- MS, TS and atrial myxoma.
- Tachycardia, hyperdynamic states, i.e. anemia, fever, thyrotoxicosis, exercise and inotropic agents.
- Shortened PR interval—Pre-excitation syndromes (i.e. Wolff-Parkinson-White [WPW] syndrome).
- Mitral valve prolapse (MVP).
- Thin individuals—S_1 can have a variable intensity in conditions that produce variable PR interval or variable ventricular contractility. This can happen in Mobitz type I heart block, digitalis toxicity, atrial fibrillation and ventricular tachycardia with AV dissociation.

Conditions associated with diminished intensity of S_1 include the followings:
- Mitral regurgitation (MR), tricuspid regurgitation (TR) and dilated cardiomyopathy.
- Prolonged PR interval (i.e. bradycardia, heart block and digitalis toxicity).
- Decreased force of ventricular contraction, i.e. cardiomyopathy, myocarditis, myxedema and myocardial infarction.
- Increased calcification of the AV valve (i.e. calcific MS and postirradiation).
- Increased distance from the heart (i.e. obesity, emphysema, pleural effusion and pericardial effusion).

Split S_1

Seen in—
- Premature ventricular contractions (PVCs) of LV origin
- Right bundle branch block
- LV pacing
- Ebstein's anomaly
- Atrial septal defect (ASD).

Reverse splitting of S_1
- This occurs when M_1 follows the closure of T_1
- This happens when the closure of mitral valve is delayed.

Conditions
- Left bundle branch block
- Right ventricular (RV) pacing
- Severe MS
- Left atrial myxoma.

Chapter 13

Second Heart Sound (S_2)

Second heart sound is produced by closure of the aortic (A_2) and pulmonary (P_2) valves.

Timing
- It occurs just after the apical impulse and carotid pulse.
- Intensity of S_2 is assessed by auscultation of aortic and pulmonary area.

Loud S_2

It may be due to either a loud A_2 or P_2, or a summation of A_2 and P_2.

Causes of Loud A_2
- Systemic hypertension
- Aortic aneurysm
- Syphilitic AR
- Atherosclerosis.

Causes of Loud P_2
- Pulmonary hypertension
- Pulmonary artery dilatation.

Soft S_2 may be Due to Soft A_2 or Soft P_2

Soft A_2
It occurs in calcific aortic stenosis.

Soft P_2
It occurs in calcific pulmonary stenosis.

Causes of delayed A_2
- Complete LBBB

- Left ventricular outflow tract obstruction
- Eisenmenger complex.

Causes of early P_2

WPW syndrome.

Table 13.1: A_2 in disease conditions

A_2	In syphilitic AR	Tambour quality
	In atherosclerotic AR	Ringing quality
	In rheumatic AR	Soft

Single S_2

Single S_2 may be either due to an absent of A_2 or P_2.

i. Absent A_2

- Aortic stenosis
- Aortic atresia.

ii. Absent P_2

- Pulmonary stenosis
- Pulmonary atresia.

Splitting of S_2

S_2 is normally split in children and young adults in inspiration.

Mechanism of Physiological Split of S_2

During inspiration, the negative intrathoracic pressure causes an increased return of blood into right ventricle causing a prolonged RV ejection time, resulting in delayed P_2.

Normal Intervals

A_2–P_2 30 milliseconds
A_2–OS   30–150 milliseconds.

Wide Split S_2

- Wide split S_2 may be variable or fixed
- Wide, variable split may be due to early A_2 or late P_2.

Early A_2

- Mitral regurgitation
- Ventricular septal defect
- Constrictive pericarditis.

Types of Split S_2 (Fig. 13.1)

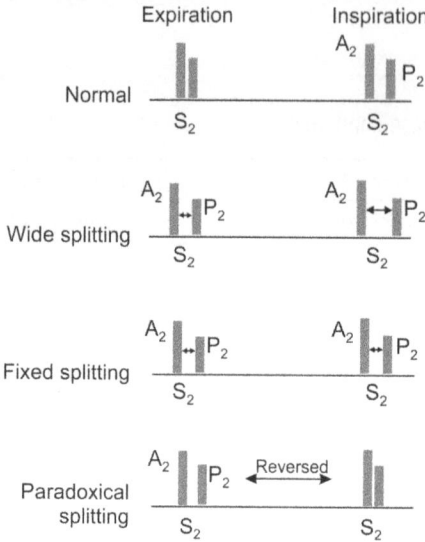

Fig. 13.1: Types of split S_2

Late P_2
- Right bundle branch block
- Left ventricular ectopics.

Wide Fixed Split
1. Atrial septal defect (ostium secundum type)
2. Partial anomalous pulmonary venous connection
3. Right ventricle failure
4. Massive acute pulmonary embolism.

In ASD, there is a wide and fixed split of S_2.

Wide splitting due to increased pulmonary hangout interval (prolonged right ventricular ejection).

Fixed splitting as the septal defect equalizes LA and RA pressures through phases of respiration.

Reverse Splitting of S_2
- Wolff-Parkinson-White (WPW) syndrome
- Aortic stenosis (severe)
- Hypertrophic cardiomyopathy
- Left bundle branch block
- Systemic hypertension.

Chapter 14

Third Heart Sound (S_3)

Introduction

- It is also known as protodiastolic sound or ventricular gallop.
- It produced by initial passive filling of the ventricles.
- Low pitch sound heard with the bell of the stethoscope.
- The presence of an S_3 is the most sensitive indicator of ventricular dysfunction.

Causes of Physiological S_3

- Children
- Young adults (< 40 years)
- Athletes
- Pregnancy.

Causes of Pathological S_3

1. High output states (anemia, pregnancy, arteriovenous fistula or thyrotoxicosis).
2. Congenital heart disease—ASD, VSD and PDA.
3. AR, MR and TR.
4. Hypertrophic cardiomyopathy.
5. Ischemic heart disease.
6. Constrictive pericarditis.
7. Systemic hypertension.
8. Pulmonary hypertension.

Table 14.1: Differentiating features between right and left ventricular S_3

Features	RV-S_3	LV-S_3
Site	Tricuspid area	Mitral area
Accentuation with respiration	On inspiration	On expiration
	Either physiological or pathological	Always pathological

Chapter 15

Fourth Heart Sound (S$_4$)

- It is also known as presystolic gallop or atrial gallop.
- It is produced by a rapid emptying of the atrium into noncompliant ventricle (late diastolic filling of the ventricle due to atrial contraction).
- A pathologic fourth heart sound usually indicates reduced ventricular compliance and impending failure.

S$_4$—Atrial Contraction Sound

It occurs shortly before the first heart sound. Although it is also called the atrial sound, and its production requires an effective atrial contraction, the fourth heart sound is the result of vibrations generated within the ventricle.

Site

- A fourth heart sound arising from the left side is best heard at the apex.
- A fourth heart sound arising from the right side is best heard at the lower-left sternal border.
- Since genesis of a fourth heart sound requires an effective atrial contraction, it does not occur in patients with atrial fibrillation.
- Physiological S$_4$ is seen in children and young adults.

Causes of Pathological S$_4$

- Hypertrophic cardiomyopathy
- Systemic hypertension
- Coronary artery disease
- Angina pectoris
- Myocardial infarction
- Ventricular aneurysm.

Gallops

Triple rhythm with tachycardia
- Triple rhythm is the presence of third heart sound
- Atrial gallop —S_1, S_2, S_4
- Ventricular gallop—S_1, S_2, S_3.

Quadruple rhythm
- Quadruple rhythm is the presence of fourth heart sound
- S_1, S_2, S_3 and S_4.

Summation gallop

Summation is the presence of S_1, S_2 with merged S_3 and S_4.

Chapter 16

Ejection Clicks

Introduction

It may be vascular or valvular.

Valvular Clicks

- Ejection clicks are produced by the opening of the semilunar valves.
- Aortic ejection click is heard in valvular aortic stenosis.
- Pulmonary ejection click is heard in valvular pulmonary stenosis.
- Pulmonary ejection click is the only right-sided event which is best heard in expiration.

Table 16.1: Differentiating features between aortic and pulmonary ejection clicks

Features	Aortic ejection click	Pulmonary ejection click
Site	Aortic area	Pulmonary area
Conduction	Heard allover precordium	Localized to pulmonary area
Accentuation	No change with respiration	Intensity increases with expiration

Midsystolic Clicks

1. Mitral valve prolapse syndrome
2. Tricuspid valve prolapse syndrome
3. Ebstein's anomaly
4. Severe AR.

Vascular Clicks

Vascular click is heard over the aortic area in—

- Aortic dilatation
- Systemic hypertension.

Vascular click is heard over the pulmonary area in—

- Pulmonary artery dilatation
- Pulmonary hypertension.

Chapter 17

Heart Murmurs

Introduction

Heart murmurs are prolonged series of auditory vibrations of variable intensity, quality and frequency. It is due to turbulence that arises when blood velocity increases due to increased flow or due to flow through a constricted or irregular orifice.

Murmurs should be described as follows—
a. Area over precordium where murmur is best heard.
b. Whether murmur is systolic or diastolic.
c. Timing and character of the murmur—early systolic murmur (ESM), pansystolic (PSM), mid-diastolic murmur (MDM) and early diastolic murmur (EDM).
d. Intensity of the murmur (grading).
e. Pitch of the murmur (lower or high-pitched).
f. Whether the murmur is best heard with the bell or the diaphragm of the stethoscope (MDM is best heard with the bell of the stethoscope, whereas ESM, EDM and PSM are best heard with the diaphragm of the stethoscope).
g. Conduction of the murmur.
h. Variation of the murmur with respiration left-sided murmurs are best heard in expiration, whereas right-sided murmurs are best heard in inspiration.
i. Posture in which murmur is best heard in the left lateral position. MDM of MS is best EDM of the AR is best heard with the patient sitting and learning forwards and holding his breath in expiration.
j. Variation of the murmur with dynamic auscultation of the murmur with, postures, pharmacological agents like amylnitrate.

Levine and Freeman's Grading of Murmurs

Systolic murmur
Grade
 1. Very soft (heard in a quiet room).

2. Soft.
3. Moderate.
4. Loud with thrill.
5. Very loud with thrill (heard with stethoscope).
6. Very loud with thrill (heard even when stethoscope is slightly away from the chest wall).

Diastolic murmur

Grade

1. Very soft
2. Soft
3. Loud
4. Loud with thrill.

Systolic Murmurs

Murmurs which occur during any part or the whole of systolic are known as systolic murmurs.

Ejection Systolic Murmurs

Causes

a. Aortic stenosis (AS)
b. Pulmonary stenosis (PS).

Table 17.1: Differentiating features between valvular AS and PS

	Features	Valvular AS	Valvular PS
1.	Site	Right 2nd intercostal space	Left 2nd intercostal space
2.	Conduction	To right carotid	To left infraclavicular area
3.	Accentuation with respiration	In expiration	In inspiration
4.	Variation of murmur with Valsalva	Murmur becomes soft	Murmur becomes loud
5.	Ejection click	No variation with respiration	Best heard over the pulmonary area during expiration
6.	P_2	----------	Soft or absent
7.	A_2	Soft or absent	--------------
8.	S_2	Reverse split	Normally or widely split

In nonvalvular aortic or pulmonary stenosis the intensity of A_2 or P_2 is normal respectively. Ejection clicks are not heard.

Late Systolic Murmurs

Causes

1. Mitral valve prolapse syndrome
2. Tricuspid valve prolapse syndrome
3. Papillary muscle dysfunction.

Pansystolic Murmurs

Causes

1. Mitral regurgitation (MR)
2. Ventricular septal defect (VSD)
3. Tricuspid regurgitation (TR).

In TR look for prominent V wave in JVP and systolic hepatic pulsation organic TR is always associated with TS. In majority of cases, TR is functional.

Table 17.2: Differentiating features among MR, TR and VSD

Features	MR	TR	VSD
Site	Apex	Left parasternal 5th or 6th intercostals space	Left parasternal 3rd or 4th intercostals space
Conduction	To axilla base and back	Localized	Localized
Accentuation with respiration	In inspiration	In inspiration	In inspiration

Diastolic Murmurs

Murmurs which occur during any part of diastolic (early, mid or late) are known as diastolic murmurs.

Early Diaslolic Murmurs (EDM)

Causes

1. AR
2. PR.

Table 17.3: Differentiating features between AR and PR

Features	AR	PR
Site	Right 2nd intercostals space and Erlis area	Left 2nd intercostals space
Accentuation with respiration	In expiration	In inspiration

Mid-diastolic Murmurs (MDM)

a. MS
b. TS.

Uncommon causes

a. Carey Coombs murmur in acute rheumatic valvulitis.
b. Austin-Flint murmur of chronic AR.
c. Acute severe AR (it is due to the diastolic flutter of the anterior mitral leaflet by the regurgitant blood stream).
d. Ritan's murmur in complete heart block.
e. Flow mid-diastolic murmurs heard in high output states.
f. Organic pulmonary regurgitation flow MDM may be heard across tricuspid valve on the right side of the heart in the following conditions.
   i. Atrial septal effect
   ii. TR
   iii. Total anomalous venous connection.

Flow MDM may be heard across the mitral value on the left side of the heart in the following conditions—

i. VSD
ii. PDA
iii. MR
iv. AR.

Late Diastolic Murmur (Presystolic Murmurs)

Causes

1. MS
2. TS
3. Atrial myxomas
4. Complete heart block.

Continuous Murmur

A continuous murmur is one that begins in systole and extends through the heart sound into part or whole of diastolic.

It is generated by flow of blood a zone of high resistance to a zone of low resistance without interruption during both systole and diastole.

Classification of Continuous Murmur

High pressure to low pressure shunts

a. Systemic to pulmonary communication patent ductus arteriosus
   - Aortopulmonary window

- Anomalous origin of left coronary artery from pulmonary artery and tricuspid atresia pulmonary atresia.
- Pulmonary AV fistula.
  b. Systemic to right-heart connection
  - Coronary arterion venous fistula
  - Rupture of sinus of Valsalva.
  c. Left atrium to right atrium connection
  - Lutembacher syndrome (ASD + acquired MS).
  d. Arteriovenous fistulae
  - Systemic
  - Pulmonary.
  e. Venovenous shunts
  - Normal flow through constricted arteries coarctation of the aorta
  - Peripheral pulmonary artery stenosis
  - Carotid stenosis
  - Celiac artery stenosis
  - Mesenteric artery stenosis
  - Renal artery stenosis.

Increased flow through normal vessels

  a. Venous (diastolic accentuation)
  - Cervical venous hum
  - Umbilical vein (Cruveilhier Baumgarten murmur)
  b. Arterial (systolic accentuation)
  - Mammary souffle
  - Uterine souffle
  - Hepatoma
  - Nephroma.

Approach to Continuous Murmurs

- Differential diagnosis when a continuous murmurs is heard
  - Presence or absence of cyanosis
  - Type of apical impulse (LV or RV)
  - Site of the murmur
  - Accentuation of the murmur (systolic or diastolic phase).

Acyanotic Heart Diseases with

1. RV type of apex
   a. Rupture or right ventricle
   b. Peripheral pulmonary artery stenosis.

2. LV type of apex
   a. Patent ductus arteriosus (PDA)
   b. Aortopulmonary window
   c. Rupture of sinus of Valsalva into the left ventricle
   d. Coronary anterior venous fistula.

Cyanotic Heart Disease with

1. RV type of apex
   - Total anomalous venous connection to SVC.
2. LV type of apex
   a. Pulmonary arteriovenous fistula
   b. Bronchopulmonary collaterals with—
      i. Tetralogy of Fallot
      ii. Tricuspid atresia
      iii. Truncus arteriosus.
3. Site of the murmur
   - In PDA continuous murmur is best heard over 1st and 2nd left intercostals spaces.
   - In aortopulmonary window, continuous murmur is best heard over the third left intercostals spaces.
   - In rupture of sinus of Valsalva continuous murmur is best heard over 3rd and 4th left intercostals spaces.

Continuous Murmur with Systolic Accentuation

1. PDA
2. Peripheral pulmonary artery stenosis.

Bronchopulmonary anastomosis

Continuous murmur with diastolic accentuation—
1. Rupture of sinus of Valsalva (RSOV).
2. Coronary arteriovenous fistula.
3. Anomalous origin of left coronary artery from pulmonary artery (ALCAPA).
4. Pulmonary arteriovenous fistula.

To and Fro Murmur (Biphasic Murmur)

A murmur is occurring through a single channel and occupying midsystolic and early diastolic and does not peak around S_2, e.g. aortic stenosis, AR, pulmonary hypertension with pulmonary regurgitation.

Table 17.4: Differentiate between continuous and to and fro murmurs

Continuous murmur	To and Fro murmur
Unidirectional	Bidirectional
S_2 engulfed by the murmur	S_2 heard well

Systolic–Diastolic Murmur

A murmur that occupies systolic and diastolic and occurs through different channels and does not peak around S_2.

Causes

VSD with AR

Table 17.5: Differentiate between PDA and VSD with AR.

Features	PDA	VSD with AR
Heart murmurs	Continuous	Systolic diastolic
Site	1st and 2nd left intercostals space	With left intercostals space
S_2	Engulfed by the murmur	Well heard
Eddy sound	Present	Absent

Innocent Murmurs

Soft systolic murmurs heard in individual without any cardiac abnormalities. They are due to increased blood flow through the ventricular outflow tracts.

They are short soft (grade 3/6 or less), systolic murmurs usually heard over supraclavicular area and along the sternal borders.

Innocent Murmurs may be Heard

1. In children, when it is known as Still's murmur.
2. In adults (> 50 years), when it is known as 50/50 murmur, i.e. 50% of adults above 50 years of age may have a systolic murmur.

Functional Murmurs

These are murmurs caused by dilation of heart chambers or vessel or increased flow.

Systolic Murmurs

Ejection systolic murmur (ESM). ESM may be heard over aortic area in—

1. Severe AR
2. Dilation of aorta.

ESM may be heard over pulmonary area in—
1. Severe PR
2. ASD
3. VSD
4. PDA
5. Dilatation of the pulmonary artery.

ESM may also be heard in certain skeletal deformities like pectus excavatum or straight back syndrome.

Pansystolic Murmur (PSM)

In dilations of LV or RV, functional PSM of mitral regurgitation (MR) or TR may be heard respectively.

Changing Murmurs

These are murmurs which change in character or intensity.
   a. Infective endocarditis
   b. Atrial thrombus
   c. Atrial myxomas.

SECTION C

Cardiovascular System and Related Diseases

18. Acute rheumatic fever (ARF)
19. Infective endocarditis
20. Mitral stenosis (MS)
21. Mitral regurgitation (MR)
22. Aortic stenosis (AS)
23. Aortic regurgitation (AR)
24. Tricuspid stenosis (TS) and tricuspid regurgitation (TR)
25. Pulmonary stenosis (PS) and pulmonary regurgitation (PR)
26. Pulmonary hypertension
27. Mitral valve prolapse (MVP)
28. Atrial septal defect (ASD)
29. Ventricular septal defect (VSD)

30. Patent ductus arteriosus (PDA)
31. Tetralogy of Fallot (TOF)
32. Eisenmenger's syndrome
33. Coarctation of the aorta
34. Other congenital heart diseases
35. Heart failure (HF)
36. Pulmonary thromboembolism (Acute cor pulmonale)
37. Cor pulmonale (Pulmonary heart disease)
38. Systemic hypertension
39. Ischemic heart disease
40. ST-segment elevation myocardial infarction (STEMI)
41. Unstable angina and non-ST-segment elevation myocardial infarction
42. Arrhythmias
43. Conduction disorders of the heart
44. Pericardial diseases
45. Myocarditis
46. Cardiomyopathy
47. Diseases of the aorta
48. Cardiac manifestations of systemic disease
49. Neoplastic diseases of the heart

Chapter 18

Acute Rheumatic Fever (ARF)

Introduction

Acute rheumatic fever (ARF) is a multisystem disease resulting from an autoimmune reaction to infection with group A β-hemolytic streptococcus. ARF and RHD are diseases of poverty. RHD is the most common cause of heart disease in children in developing countries.

Epidemiology

ARF is mainly a disease of children aged 5–14 years. Prevalence of RHD peaks between 25 and 40 years. RHD more commonly affects females. It is rare before 4 years and after 40 years.

Pathogenesis

ARF is exclusively caused by infection of the upper respiratory tract with group A streptococci. It is now thought that any strain of group A streptococcus has the potential to cause ARF.

It is currently thought that the initial damage is due to cross-reactive antibodies attaching at the cardiac valve endothelium, leading to subsequent T cell-mediated inflammation.

Clinical Features

There is a latent period of 3 weeks between the precipitating group A streptococcal infection and the appearance of the clinical features of ARF. The exceptions are chorea and carditis, which may follow prolonged latent periods lasting upto 6 months. The preceding group A streptococcal infection is commonly subclinical. The most common clinical presentation of ARF is polyarthritis and fever. Polyarthritis is present in 60–75% of cases and carditis in 50–60%. Chorea is present in upto 30% of cases. Erythema marginatum and subcutaneous nodules are now rare.

Heart Involvement

- Upto 60% of patients with ARF progress to RHD
- The endocardium, pericardium, or myocardium may be affected
- Valvular damage is the hallmark of rheumatic carditis.

The mitral valve is almost always affected, sometimes together with the aortic valve; isolated aortic valve involvement is rare.

The characteristic manifestation of carditis is mitral regurgitation

Over years, usually as a result of recurrent episodes, leaflet thickening, scarring, calcification and valvular stenosis may develop.

Myocardial inflammation may affect electrical conduction pathways, leading to first-degree AV block and softening of the first heart sound.

Joint Involvement

It is migratory polyarthritis. ARF almost always affects the large joints—most commonly the knees, ankles, hips and elbows—and it is asymmetric.

Chorea

Sydenham's chorea—It follows a prolonged latent period after group A streptococcal infection is found mainly in females.

The choreiform movements affect particularly the head (causing characteristic darting movements of the tongue) and the upper limbs.

Skin Manifestations

Erythema marginatum (Fig. 18.1)

It begins as pink macules that clear centrally, leaving a serpiginous and spreading edge.

It occurs usually on the trunk, sometimes on the limbs, but almost never on the face.

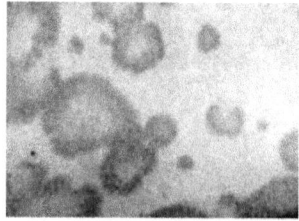

Fig. 18.1: Eythema marginatum

Subcutaneous Nodules (Fig. 18.2)

- Occur as painless.
- Small (0.5–2 cm).
- Nodules on the hands, feet, elbows, occiput and rarely on the vertebra.
- They are a delayed manifestation, appearing 2–3 weeks after the onset of disease.
- Last for 1–3 weeks.
- Commonly associated with carditis.

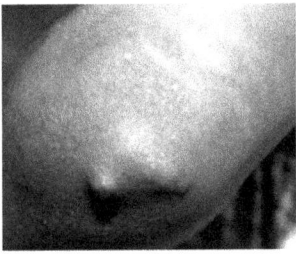

Fig. 18.2: Subcutaneous nodules

Other Features

- Fever occurs in most cases of ARF.
- High-grade fever.
- Elevated acute-phase reactants—CRP and ESR are often dramatically elevated.
- Leukocytosis is seen.
- Evidence of a preceding group A streptococcal infection.
- It is essential in making the diagnosis of ARF. The most common serologic tests are the antistreptolysin O (ASO) and anti-DNase B (ADB) titers.

Confirming the Diagnosis

Criteria first proposed by Dr T Duckett Jones in 1944 and modified by WHO in 1992.

1992 revised Jones criteria

Major manifestations	Carditis Polyarthritis Chorea Erythema marginatum Subcutaneous nodules
Minor manifestations	Clinical: Fever, polyarthralgia Laboratory: Elevated ESR or leukocyte count ECG: Prolonged P-R interval

Contd...

Contd...

Essential criteria—Supporting evidence of a preceding streptococcal infection within the last 45 days	Elevated ASO titer (>333 todd units in children, >250 todd units in adults) or A positive throat culture, or Rapid antigen test for group A streptococcus, or Recent scarlet fever

Two major or one major and two minor criteria, in the presence of essential criteria is required to diagnose acute rheumatic fever.

- **Treatment**: Acute rheumatic fever.

Investigations
White blood cell count
Erythrocyte sedimentation rate
C-reactive protein
Blood cultures if febrile
Electrocardiogram
Echocardiogram
Throat swab culture for group A streptococcus
Antistreptococcal serology: Both antistreptolysin O and anti D Nase B titers.

Antibiotics

Penicillin is the drug of choice can be given orally—Phenoxymethyl penicillin 500 mg twice daily, or amoxicillin 50 mg/kg, for 10 days or as a single dose of 1.2 million IM benzathine penicillin G.

Salicylates

Aspirin is the drug of choice. An initial dose of 100 mg/kg/day in 4 divided doses is given for upto 2 weeks.

Glucocorticoids

The use of glucocorticoids remains controversial.

Treatment of carditis (causing heart failure) with glucocorticoids reduce the acute inflammation and result in more rapid resolution of failure.

Prednisolone are recommended at doses of 1–2 mg/kg/day upto a maximum of 3 weeks.

Bed rest

Bed rest should be prescribed for arthritis and arthralgia and for patients with heart failure.

Chorea

Treat with carbamazepine or sodium valproate.

Prevention

The mainstay of controlling ARF and RHD is secondary prevention (Table 18.1).

Benzathine penicillin G 1.2 million units every 4 weeks. It can be given every 3 weeks to persons at high-risk.

Oral penicillin V (250 mg) can be given twice daily, instead, but is somewhat less effective than benzathine penicillin G.

Penicillin-allergic patients can receive erythromycin (250 mg) twice daily.

Table 18.1: Duration of prophylaxis for secondary prevention of ARF

Category of patient	Duration of prophylaxis
Rheumatic fever without carditis	For 5 years after the last attack or 21 years of age (whichever is longer)
Rheumatic fever with carditis but no residual valvular disease	For 10 years after the last attack, or 21 years of age (whichever is longer)
Rheumatic fever with persistent valvular disease, evident clinically or on echocardiography	For 10 years after the last attack, or 40 years of age (whichever is longer). Sometimes lifelong prophylaxis

Chapter 19

Infective Endocarditis

Introduction

The prototypic lesion of infective endocarditis is the vegetation. Infection most commonly involves heart valves (either native or prosthetic) in VSD or on intracardiac devices themselves. The analogous process involving arteriovenous shunts, patent ductus arteriosus, or a coarctation of the aorta is called infective endarteritis.

Acute Endocarditis

- Hectically febrile illness
- Rapidly damages cardiac structures
- Hematogenously seeds extracardiac sites
- If untreated, progresses to death within weeks.

Subacute Endocarditis

Follows an indolent course causes structural cardiac damage only slowly rarely metastasizes is gradually progressive unless complicated by a major embolic event or ruptured mycotic aneurysm.

Etiology

- Streptococci
- Pneumococci
- Enterococci
- *Staphylococcus aureus*
- Coagulase-negative staphylococci
- Fastidious gram-negative coccobacilli (HACEK group)
- Gram-negative bacilli
- Candida spp
- Polymicrobial/miscellaneous

- Diphtheroids
- Culture-negative.

The oral cavity, skin and upper respiratory tract are the respective primary portals for the viridans streptococci, staphylococci and HACEK (haemophilus, actinobacillus, cardiobacterium, eikenella and kingella) organisms.

Prosthetic Valve Endocarditis (PVE)

Arising within 2 months of valve surgery is generally nosocomial, *Staphylococcus aureus*, coagulase negative streptococci, facultative gram-negative bacilli, diphtheroids and fungi.

Transvenous pacemaker or implanted defibrillator-associated endocarditis is usually nosocomial.

Endocarditis Occurring Among Injection Drug Users

Involves the tricuspid valve, is commonly caused by MRSA.

From 5–15% of patients with endocarditis have negative blood cultures.

In one-third to one-half of these cases, cultures are negative because of prior antibiotic exposure.

Pathogenesis

Endothelial injury allows either direct infection by virulent organisms or the development of an uninfected platelet-fibrin thrombus—A condition called nonbacterial thrombotic endocarditis (NBTE).

The cardiac conditions most commonly resulting in NBTE are mitral regurgitation, aortic stenosis, aortic regurgitation, ventricular septal defects and complex congenital heart disease.

NBTE also arises as a result of a hypercoagulable state—Marantic endocarditis (uninfected vegetations seen in patients with malignancy and chronic diseases).

Clinical Manifestations

The clinical syndrome of infective endocarditis is highly variable and spans a continuum between acute and subacute presentations.

Hemolytic streptococci, *Staphylococcus aureus* and pneumococci typically result in an acute course, subacute endocarditis is typically caused by viridans streptococci, enterococci, CoNS and the HACEK group.

Clinical Features (Fig. 19.1)

- Fever.
- Chills and sweats.

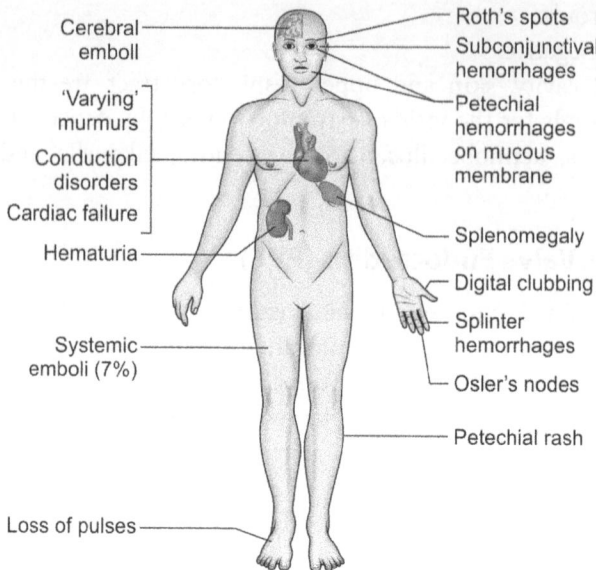

Fig. 19.1: Clinical manifestations of infective endocarditis

- Anorexia, weight loss and malaise.
- Myalgias and arthralgias.
- Back pain.
- Heart murmur.
- New/worsened regurgitant murmur.
- Arterial emboli.
- Splenomegaly.
- Clubbing.
- Neurologic manifestations.
- Peripheral manifestations (Osler's nodes, splinter hemorrhages, Janeway lesions and Roth's spots).
- Petechiae.
- Laboratory manifestations.
  - Anemia
  - Leukocytosis
  - Microscopic hematuria
  - Elevated erythrocyte sedimentation rate
  - Elevated C-reactive protein level
  - Rheumatoid factor
  - Circulating immune complexes
  - Decreased serum complement.

In patients with subacute presentations, fever is typically low-grade.

Cardiac Manifestations

Although heart murmurs are usually indicative of the predisposing cardiac pathology rather than of endocarditis, valvular damage and ruptured chordae may result in new regurgitant murmurs.

Congestive heart failure (CHF) develops in 30–40% of patients.
Emboli to a coronary artery occur in 2% of patients and may result in myocardial infarction.

Septic embolization is common in patients with acute *Staphylococcus aureus* endocarditis.

Hematogenously seeded focal infection is evident in the skin, spleen, kidneys, skeletal system and meninges.

Arterial emboli are clinically apparent in upto 50% of patients.

Cerebrovascular emboli presenting as strokes, encephalopathy complicate 30% of cases of endocarditis. Other neurologic complications are aseptic or purulent meningitis, intracranial hemorrhage, abscess and seizures.

Renal Manifestation

Immune complex deposition on the glomerular basement membrane causes diffuse hypocomplementemic glomerulonephritis and renal dysfunction.

Embolic renal infarcts may occur.

Diagnosis

The Duke criteria.

Duke criteria—It has been developed on the basis of clinical, laboratory and echocardiographic findings (Table 19.1).

Documentation

- Of two major criteria
- Of one major criterion and three minor criteria
- Of five minor criteria allows a clinical diagnosis of definite endocarditis.

Table 19.1: The Duke criteria

The Duke criteria for the clinical diagnosis of infective endocarditis
Major criteria
1. Positive blood culture
2. Evidence of endocardial involvement
Positive echocardiogram

Contd...

Contd...

Abscess, or
New valvular regurgitation
3. Blood cultures drawn >12 hours apart
Minor criteria
1. Predisposition: Predisposing heart condition or injection drug use 2. Fever: 38.0°C 3. Vascular phenomena: Major arterial emboli, septic pulmonary infarcts, mycotic aneurysm, intracranial hemorrhage, conjunctival hemorrhages and Janeway lesions 4. Immunologic phenomena: Glomerulonephritis, Osler's nodes, Roth's spots and rheumatoid factor 5. Microbiologic evidence: Positive blood culture but not meeting major criterion as noted previously or serologic evidence of active infection with organism consistent with infective endocarditis

Definite endocarditis is defined by documentation of two major criteria, of one major criterion and three minor criteria, or of five minor criteria.

Transesophageal echocardiography is recommended for assessing possible prosthetic valve endocarditis.

Blood cultures

Echocardiography

Transthoracic echocardiography (TTE) is noninvasive and exceptionally specific.

Treatment: Infective endocarditis
- Antimicrobial therapy
- Penicillin G (2–3 mU IV q4 hourly for 4 weeks)
- Ceftriaxone (2 gm/d IV as a single dose for 4 weeks)
- Vancomycin (15 mg/kg IV q12 hourly for 4 weeks)
- Monitoring antimicrobial therapy
- Blood cultures should be repeated till culture is sterile
- Surgical treatment is also indicated.

Prevention

Antibiotic regimens for prophylaxis of endocarditis in adults with high-risk cardiac lesions
A. Standard oral regimen
1. Amoxicillin: 2 gm per orally 1 hour before procedure

If allergic, third generation cephalosporin, clindamycin and azithromycin may be given.

Chapter 20

Mitral Stenosis (MS)

Etiology
- Rheumatic fever is the most common cause
- Congenital-parachute mitral valve
- Mitral annular calcification
- SLE and RA
- Left atrial myxoma
- Infective endocarditis with large vegetations
- Hunter's syndrome
- Hurler's syndrome
- Carcinoid syndrome
- Drug—Methysergide
- Amyloidosis.

Pure or predominant mitral stenosis occurs in approximately 40% of all patients with rheumatic heart.

Pathology
In rheumatic mitral stenosis, the valve leaflets are diffusely thickened by fibrous tissue and/or calcific deposits. The mitral commissures fuse, the chordae tendineae fuse and shorten, the valvular cusps become rigid, and lead to narrowing of the funnel-shaped ("fish-mouth") valve.

Thrombus formation may arise from the calcific valve itself, but in patients with atrial fibrillation (AF), thrombi arise more frequently from the dilated left atrium (LA), particularly from within the left atrial appendage.

Pathophysiology
- In normal adults, the area of the mitral valve orifice is 4–6 cm^2
- Valve area >2.5 cm^2—No symptoms
- Mild mitral stenosis—1.5–2.5 cm^2
- Moderate mitral stenosis—1–1.5 cm^2

- Severe /critical mitral stenosis < 1cm^2
- Pinhole mitral stenosis < 0.5 cm^2.

Juvenile Mitral Stenosis

- Usually found in India
- Below 18 years
- AF and valve calcification rare
- Pinpoint mitral valve
- Needs immediate surgery.

Pulmonary Hypertension

Pulmonary hypertension results from:
1. Passive backward transmission of the elevated left atrium pressure.
2. Pulmonary arteriolar constriction.
   Pulmonary hypertension results in right ventricle enlargement, secondary tricuspid regurgitation (TR) and pulmonic regurgitation (PR), as well as right-sided heart failure.

Symptoms

The latent period between the initial attack of rheumatic carditis and the development of symptoms due to mitral stenosis is generally about two decades.

Exertional dyspnea may be precipitated by sudden changes in the heart rate, severe exertion, excitement, fever, severe anemia, paroxysmal atrial fibrillation, pregnancy and thyrotoxicosis. As mitral stenosis progresses, orthopnea and paroxysmal nocturnal dyspnea develop.

Symptoms begin in 4th decade but earlier in developing countries.

Palpitation
- Fatigue
- Recurrent bronchitis.

Hemoptysis

Causes
- Pulmonary apoplexy—Rupture of pulmonary-bronchial venous connections.
- Pink frothy sputum of pulmonary edema.
- Recurrent bronchitis.
- Pulmonary infarction.
- Pulmonary hemosiderosis.
- Anticoagulation therapy.

Atrial Fibrillation (AF)
- Occurs in 2/3rd of patients with mitral stenosis.
- Atrial fibrillation more common in mitral stenosis than mitral regurgitation.
- Pulse is irregularly irregular, absent a waves in JVP and varying intensity of S_1.
- Atrial fibrillation precipitates CCF and thromboembolic episodes.
- Systemic emboli occurs.

Pulmonary Edema

It occurs in severe mitral stenosis due to left atrium failure. Less common in long standing mitral stenosis due to thickened alveolar capillary membrane.

Infective endocarditis more common in mitral stenosis with associated mitral regurgitation.

Chest Pain
- Anginal pain may be due to coincidental coronary atherosclerosis or secondary to coronary embolization.

Pressure Symptoms
a. Compression of left recurrent laryngeal nerve by enlarged left atrium results in hoarseness of voice (Ortner's syndrome).
b. Compression of esophagus by enlarged left atrium causes dysphagia.

Physical Findings
- Mitral facies—Malar flush with blue facies.
- Small volume pulse.
- In patients with sinus rhythm and severe pulmonary hypertension, the jugular venous pulse reveals prominent 'a' waves.
- Blood pressure is usually normal or slightly low.
- Left parasternal heave present.
- Tapping apical impulse (palpable S_1).
- A diastolic thrill at the cardiac apex, with the patient in the left lateral position.

Auscultation

The first heart sound (S_1) is loud.

Cause

Due to persistent diastolic gradient across mitral valve, valve cusps remain wide open throughout diastole and as soon as ventricular systole starts, the wide opened valve cusps close rapidly, giving rise to loud S_1.

The pulmonic component of the second heart sound (P_2) also is often loud.

The opening snap (OS) of the mitral valve is most readily audible in expiration at, or just medial to, the cardiac apex. Opening snap follows A_2 by 0.05–0.12 s. The time interval between A_2 and opening snap varies inversely with the severity of the mitral stenosis. Opening snap indicates pliability of the valve. Opening snap is also audible in TS.

A low-pitched, rough and rumbling, mid-diastolic murmur with presystolic accentuation, heard best at the apex with the bell of the sthethoscope, patient in the left lateral recumbent position in expiration. It is accentuated by mild exercise (a few rapid sit-ups) carried out just before auscultation. The duration of this murmur correlates with the severity of the stenosis. presystolic accentuation is absent in atrial fibrillation.

Systolic murmurs of functional mitral regurgitation may be heard at the apex in pure mitral stenosis.

Hepatomegaly, ankle edema, ascites, and pleural effusion, particularly in the right pleural cavity, may occur in patients with mitral stenosis and right ventricular failure (RV).

Associated Lesions

With severe pulmonary hypertension, a pansystolic murmur produced by functional tricuspid regurgitation may be audible along the left sternal border. This murmur is usually louder during inspiration and diminishes during forced expiration (Carvallo's sign).

When the cardiac output is markedly reduced in mitral stenosis, the typical auscultatory findings, including the diastolic rumbling murmur, may not be detectable (silent mitral stenosis).

The Graham Steell murmur of pulmonary regurgitation, a high-pitched, diastolic, decrescendo blowing murmur along the left sternal border occurs in mitral stenosis with severe pulmonary hypertension.

ECG (Fig. 20.1)

- In mitral stenosis and sinus rhythm, inverted P due to left atrial overload.
- P mitrale (bifid P) in lead 2 when left atrial (LA) enlargement occurs.
- The QRS complex is usually normal.
- With severe pulmonary hypertension, right-axis deviation and RVH.

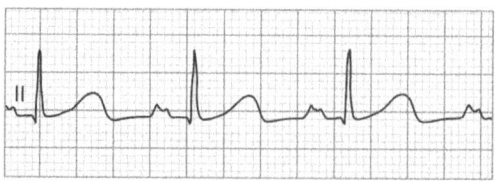

Fig. 20.1: P mitrale

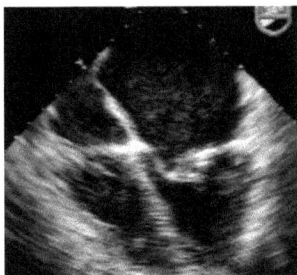

Fig. 20.2: Echo in MS

Echocardiogram (Fig. 20.2)

Transthoracic echocardiography (TTE) with color Doppler imaging is the investigation of choice.

Thickened immobile cusps; reduced rate of diastolic filling; reduced valve area.

Chest X-ray (Fig. 20.3)

Straightening of the left border of heart (due to prominent pulmonary artery and left atrial appendage). Shadow within shadow—Double shadow behind the heart in right heart border—Left atrial enlargement prominence of the main pulmonary arteries dilation of the upper lobe pulmonary veins posterior displacement of the esophagus by an enlarged left atrium (LA).

Kerley B lines are fine, horizontal lines in the lower and mid-lung fields that result from interlobular lymphatic edema when LA pressure exceeds 20 mmHg.
- Later, mitral valve calcification
  - Kerley A lines (Straight, dense lines upto 4 cm in length and running towards the hilum when pulmonary venous pressure is more than 30 mmHg).
- Rarely, findings of pulmonary hemosiderosis and parenchymal ossification.

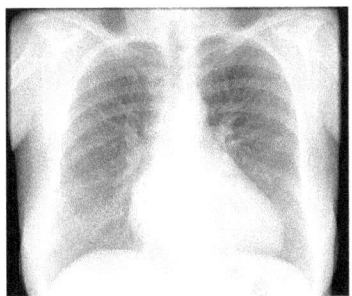

Fig. 20.3: Chest X-ray findings in MS

Barium swallow in right anterior oblique (RAO) view—Sickling of barium filled esophagus due to compression by enlarged LA.

Differential Diagnosis

1. Functional—mid-diastolic murmur at apex in isolated mitral regurgitation.
2. The apical mid-diastolic murmur associated with severe AR (Austin-Flint murmur).
3. Left atrial myxoma.
4. Cor triatriatum.
5. Ball valve thrombus of left atrium.
6. Carey-Coombs murmur of mitral valvulitis.

Atrial Myxoma

It may present with fever, anemia, weight loss and systemic emboli.

Cardiac Catheterization

Catheterization and left ventriculography are indicated in patients who have undergone mitral valvotomy.

Treatment

Mitral stenosis.

Medical treatment

- β-blockers, nondihydropyridine calcium channel blockers, or digoxin for rate control of atrial fibrillation.
- Cardioversion for new-onset atrial fibrillation and HF.
- Diuretics for HF.
- Warfarin for atrial fibrillation or thromboembolism.

Penicillin prophylaxis for secondary prevention of rheumatic fever

- Benzathine penicillin 1.2 million units deep IM every 3 weeks.
- Oral penicillin 800 mg once daily may also be given.
- Rheumatic fever without carditis—Minimum 5 years or upto 20 years of life, whichever is greater.
- Rheumatic fever with carditis—Lifelong prophylaxis.
- Infective endocarditis prophylaxis.

Mitral valvotomy

Mitral valvotomy is indicated in symptomatic patients with isolated mitral stenosis, whose effective orifice <1.5 cm^2. Mitral valvotomy can be carried out by two techniques: Percutaneous mitral balloon valvotomy (closed) and surgical valvotomy (open).

Percutaneous balloon valvuloplasty

Mitral valve replacement (MVR)
- Mitral stenosis with significant mitral regurgitation.
- Those in whom the valve has been severely distorted by previous transcatheter or operative manipulation.

Mechanical Prosthesis
  a. Caged ball valve (Starr-Edwards prosthesis)
  b. Tilting-disk valve (St Jude, Bjork-Shiley valves).

Bioprosthesis
  a. Porcine bioprosthesis
  b. Pericardial xenograft prosthesis.

Chapter 21

Mitral Regurgitation (MR)

Mitral Regurgitation (Fig. 21.1)

Causes

- Rheumatic heart disease.
- Congenital mitral regurgitation [parachute mitral valve, endocardial cushion defects (in ostium primum ASD) and mitral valve prolapsed syndrome].
- Infective endocarditis.
- Ischemic heart disease (papillary muscle dysfunction and rupture).
- Dilated cardiomyopathy.
- Traumatic.
- Following cardiac surgery.
  - Amyloidosis.
  - Sarcoidosis.

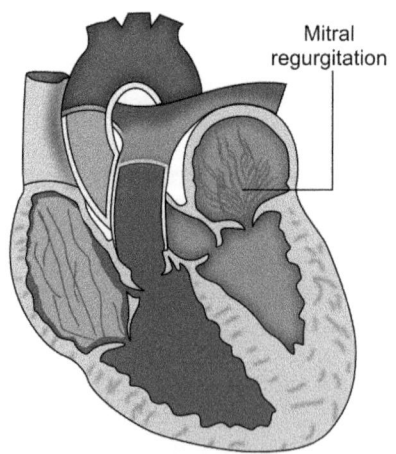

Fig. 21.1: Mitral regurgitation

- Connective tissue disorders
  1. Ankylosing spondylitis
  2. Rheumatoid arthritis
  3. Systemic lupus erythematosus
  4. Marfan's syndrome
  5. Ehlers-Danlos syndrome.

Acute MR can occur in the setting of acute myocardial infarction (MI) with papillary muscle rupture, following blunt chest wall trauma, or during the course of infective endocarditis.

Causes of Acute MR

- Infective endocarditis.
- Trauma.
- Acute rheumatic fever.
- Myocardial infarction (rupture of papillary muscle specially in inferior wall MI).
- Myocardial abscess.
- Connective tissue disorders.
- Myxomatous degeneration of the valve.

Symptoms

- Exertional dyspnea, fatigue and palpitation.
- Sudden onset of dyspnea, PND, orthopnea in acute MR.

Signs

Pulse

1. Normal in mild mitral regurgitation (MR).
2. Hyperkinetic in moderate to severe MR—Quick rising with normal volume (small water hammer pulse or pseudocollapsing pulse).

- Wide pulse pressure.
- Hyperdynamic apical impulse which is shifted down and out left parasternal heave.
- Soft S_1.
- LV S_3.
- P_2 loud and S_2 widely split in pulmonary hypertension (widely split S_2 is due to premature aortic valve closure).
- S_4 is heard only in acute MR.
- Systolic thrill over mitral area.
- A pansystolic murmur at apex, radiating to axilla and back if anterior leaflet is involved or to base if posterior leaflet is involved. MR murmur

(not due to MVP) is increased by hand grip and decreased during straining phase of Valsalva.

Seagull Murmur or Cooing Dove Murmur
- Seen in acute myocardial infarction and infective endocarditis in MR.
- Musical quality of murmur due to rupture chordae tendinae acting as string of musical instrument.

Signs of AF
- AF is better tolerated and less common in mitral regurgitation than in MS.
- A systolic murmur heard over the apex may be either due to MR or aortic stenosis. With the development of AF, systolic murmur of AS changes from beat to beat whereas murmur of MR remains unchanged.

Severity
The following indicate severity of MR is:
- Presence of systolic thrill over apex
- Large LV indicates severe MR
- Presence of S_3
- Flow MDM across nonstenotic mitral valve indicates severe MR.

Complications
1. Atrial fibrillation
2. Thromboembolism
3. Infective endocarditis (more common than in MS)
4. Cardiac failure.

ECG
- LA overload
- LV enlargement
- Atrial fibrillation.

Chest X-ray
1. Cardiomegaly (due to left atrial, left ventricular and later right ventricular enlargement).
2. Calcification of annulus or leaflets.
3. Signs of pulmonary venous hypertension and pulmonary edema.

Echocardiogram
1. Dilated LA (giant or aneurysmal left atrium) and LV

2. Dynamic LV
3. Regurgitation detectable.

Cardiac Catheterization

- Dilated LA and LV
- Mitral regurgitation
- Pulmonary hypertension may be present.

Management

Medical

1. Same as for MS.
2. ACE inhibitors are useful in the treatment of chronic MR.
3. Intravenous nitroprusside or nitroglycerine reduce the afterload and thereby the volume of regurgitant flow and thus useful in stabilizing patients with acute and or severe MR.
4. Diuretics and intra-aortic counter pulsation are useful in acute MR.

Surgical

- Indication for surgery—LV end-systolic dimension of > 45 mm or LVEF < 60% denotes severe LV dysfunction.
- Surgery is indicated when there is progressive deterioration in LV function despite antifailure measures.
- Plastic reparative procedure of mitral valve (in young patients).
- Valve replacement in older patients.

Surgery for acute MR

1. Failure of medical therapy to stabilize the patient in acute MR
2. Emergency surgery is indicated in case of papillary muscle rupture.

Chapter 22

Aortic Stenosis (AS)

Introduction

Aortic stenosis occurs in about one-fourth of all patients with chronic valvular heart disease; approximately 80% of adult patients with symptomatic valvular aortic stenosis are male.

Common Causes

1. Congenital aortic stenosis (supravalvular aortic stenosis, valvular aortic stenosis and subvalvular aortic stenosis).
2. Rheumatic aortic stenosis.
3. Degenerative (senile) calcific aortic stenosis.
4. Atherosclerotic aortic stenosis (common after 65 years).

Patients with rheumatic aortic stenosis almost always have concomitant mitral valve involvement. Rheumatic disease of the aortic leaflets produces commissural fusion.

The presence of aortic valve sclerosis (focal thickening and calcification of the leaflets not severe enough to cause obstruction) is associated with an excess risk of cardiovascular death and myocardial infarction among persons older than age 65. Approximately 30% of persons older than 65 years exhibit aortic valve sclerosis.

Normal aortic valve area is 3–4 cm^2.

Bicuspid Aortic Valve Disease

A bicuspid aortic valve is the most common congenital heart valve defect and occurs in 0.5–1.4% of the population with male to female predominance. The inheritance pattern appears to be autosomal dominant with incomplete penetrance.

Williams syndrome is supravalvular aortic stenosis with "elfin" facies and transient hypercalcemia.

Shone's syndrome (Shone's complex) is congenital heart disease with parachute mitral valve, subaortic stenosis and coarctation of the aorta.

Symptoms

Aortic stenosis is rarely of clinical importance until the valve orifice has narrowed to approximately 1 cm². Even severe aortic stenosis may exist for many years without producing any symptoms because of the ability of the hypertrophied LV to generate the elevated intraventricular pressures required to maintain a normal stroke volume. Once symptoms occur, valve replacement is indicated.

Exertional dyspnea, angina pectoris, and syncope are the three cardinal symptoms.

Orthopnea, paroxysmal nocturnal dyspnea, and pulmonary edema, i.e. symptoms of LV failure, also occur only in the advanced stages of the disease. Severe pulmonary hypertension leading to RV failure and systemic venous hypertension, hepatomegaly, AF, and TR are usually late findings in patients with isolated severe aortic stenosis.

When aortic stenosis and mitral stenosis coexist, the reduction in cardiac output induced by mitral stenosis lowers the pressure gradient across the aortic valve and, thereby, masks many of the clinical findings produced by AS.

Signs

- Slow rising, small volume pulse—Pulsus parvus et. tardus.
- Combined AS, AR—Pulsus bisferiens is seen.
- Bernheim effect—In many patients, the 'a' wave in the jugular venous pulse is accentuated. This results from the diminished distensibility of the RV cavity caused by the bulging, hypertrophied interventricular septum.

Apex

1. Heaving apex beat.
2. The LV impulse is usually displaced laterally.
3. A double apical impulse (with a palpable S_4) may be present with the patient in the left lateral recumbent position.

- A systolic thrill may be present at the aortic area when leaning forward.
- Carotid thrill (shudder)—A thrill or anacrotic "shudder" may be palpable over the carotid arteries, more commonly the left.
- S_4 may be heard.
- Ejection click—It indicates valvular AS and disappears on calcification of aortic valve.

- A rough, grunting, ejection (mid) systolic murmur loudest in the aortic area. It is characteristically low-pitched, rough and rasping in character. It is transmitted upward along the carotid arteries.
- Occasionally it is transmitted downward along 2nd aortic area and to the apex (Gallavardin effect).

Severity

1. According to S_2
   - Mild stenosis—A_2 followed by P_2
   - Moderate stenosis—A_2 is delayed giving rise to single S_2
   - Severe stenosis—Reverse splitting of $S_2(P_2-A_2)$.
2. According to valve area
   - In severe AS, valve area is < 0.75 cm²/m² body surface area.
   - In critical AS, valve area is < 0.5 cm²/m² body surface area.
3. Long murmur, loud murmur and late peaking of murmur indicate severe AS.
4. According to the gradient across aortic valve
   Normal gradient—0 mmHg
   Stenotic gradient—
   - Mild AS < 25 mmHg
   - Moderate AS 25–40 mmHg
   - Severe AS > 40 mmHg.
5. Presence of S_4 and absent A_2 indicate severe AS.
6. Presence of S_3 in AS means severe systolic dysfunction and elevated filling pressure.

Silent AS

1. Severe AS with CCF (low cardiac output).
   In this situation, AS murmur is not heard. But murmur reappears on treating failure.
2. When MS is associated with AS usually MS masks the signs of AS.

Complications

1. Left ventricular failure
2. Arrhythmias including sudden death
3. Complete heart block
4. Infective endocarditis
5. Gastrointestinal bleed due to angiodysplasia of colon.

Investigations

ECG
- LVH with strain pattern.
- LBBB, complete heart block if calcification of valve extends into the conducting system.

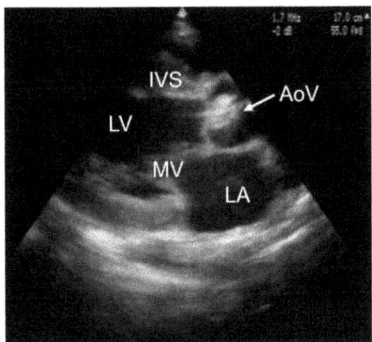

Fig. 22.1: Echo findings in AS

Chest X-ray
- Poststenotic dilatation of ascending aorta in valvular AS
- Calcification of aortic valve on lateral view.

Echocardiogram (Fig. 22.1)
1. Calcified valve
2. Hypertrophied LV
3. Doppler estimate of gradient.

Cardiac catheterization
1. Systolic gradient between LV and aorta
2. Poststenotic dilatation of aorta
3. Regurgitation of aortic valve may be present.

Coronary angiogram
- To rule out coronary artery disease only in patients with AS developing symptoms of angina.
- It is indicated in patients > 45 years with severe AS.

Prognosis
Average life expectancy after the onset of various symptoms is as follows:
- Angina—3 years
- Syncope—3 years

- Dyspnea—2 years
- Heart failure—2 years.

Management

Medical

- Treatment of cardiac failure.
- Rheumatic fever prophylaxis.
- Infective endocarditis prophylaxis.
- Use diuretics with caution to avoid volume depletion in the management of cardiac failure.
- ACE inhibitors should be avoided in moderate or severe aortic stenosis.
- Nitroglycerine is useful for the relief of angina.
- Statins are useful in the management of degenerative calcific aortic stenosis.

Surgical

- Aortic valve replacement (AVR)—When systolic gradient across the valve is > 40 mmHg and when there is progressive LV dysfunction. In patients without heart failure, the operative risk of AVR is approximately 3%. Prior to AVR, coronary angiogram is done to detect coronary occlusion.
- If patient is unfit for surgery, percutaneous, transluminal aortic valvuloplasty can be tried. It is also useful in children and young adults with congenital AS, and also as a bridge to surgery in patients with severe LV dysfunction.
- Simple commissural incision under direct vision is done in children and adolescents with noncalcific congenital AS.
- Percutaneous aortic valve replacement.

Chapter 23
Aortic Regurgitation (AR)

Causes: AR may be caused by primary valve disease or by primary aortic root disease.

Aortic Valve Involvement

1. Rheumatic heart disease
2. Infective endocarditis
3. Congenital bicuspid aortic valve
4. Secondary AR in subaortic stenosis.

Primary Aortic Root Disease

1. Syphilis
2. Ankylosing spondylitis
3. Marfan's syndrome
4. Ehlers-Danlos syndrome
5. Aortic dissection
6. Systemic hypertension
7. Osteogenesis imperfecta
8. Idiopathic dilatation of aorta
9. Annuloaortic ectasia.

Causes of acute AR

- Infective endocarditis
- Aortic dissection
- Trauma.

Symptoms

1. Exertional dyspnea
2. Palpitation
3. Angina (in severe AR).

Severe acute AR may present as pulmonary edema and/or cardiogenic shock.

Chronic severe AR may have a long latent period, and patients may remain relatively asymptomatic for as long as 10–15 years.

Peripheral Signs of AR—Signs of Wide Pulse Pressure

1. **Lighthouse sign**—Alternate flushing and blanching of forehead.
2. **Landolfi's sign**—Change in pupillary size in accordance with cardiac cycle.
3. **Becker's sign**—Retinal artery pulsations.
4. **De Musset's sign**—Head nodding with each heartbeat.
5. **Müller's sign**—Pulsatile uvula.
6. **Quincke's sign**—Capillary pulsations can be detected by pressing a glass slide on lip or nail bed.
7. **Corrigan's sign**—Dancing carotids.
8. **Locomotor brachii**—Dancing brachials.
9. **Watson's Water-Hammer or collapsing pulse or pulsus celer**—It is a large volume pulse. There is a rapid upstroke and rapid downstroke. Systolic pressure is high and diastolic pressure is low.
   Corrigan's pulse—Quick collapse of carotid pulse in AR.
   (Water-hammer toy is a sealed glass tube partly filled with water, which when shaken produces the sound of impact of a hammer).
10. **Bisferiens pulse**—In severe AR or combined AS or AR.
11. **Traube's sign**—Pistol shot femorals.
12. **Duroziez's sign**—Systolic murmur heard over femoral artery when it is compressed proximally and a diastolic murmur when it is compressed distally using the 'bell' of the stethoscope.
    Duroziez's murmur—Diastolic murmur heard with the diaphragm of the stethoscope when distal pressure is applied.
13. **Hill's sign**—Lower limb systolic pressure exceeds brachial pressure by > 20 mmHg.
    - Mild AR 20–40 mmHg
    - Moderate AR 40–60 mmHg
    - Severe AR > 60 mmHg.
14. **Rosenbach's sign**—Pulsations of liver.
15. **Gerhardt's sign**—Pulsations over enlarged spleen.
16. **Maynes sign**—A drop of 15 mmHg in diastolic blood pressure on raising the arm.

Other signs

- Apical impulse is displaced downwards and outwards (due to LV enlargement) and hyperdynamic (forcible) in nature.

- Soft S_1—Only in acute AR.
- S_3 may be heard.

Murmur

1. A high pitch decresendo early diastolic murmur immediately after A_2, best heard in left 3rd or 4th sternal border with the diaphragm of the stethoscope with the patient sitting up, leaning forwards, breath in expiration.
2. Flow ESM across aortic valve heard at aortic area, conducted to carotids.
3. Flow MDM across mitral valve—Austin-Flint murmur—(mechanism-Regurgitant blood stream impinging upon the anterior leaflet of mitral valve).

- AR murmur in aortic area—Aortic root dilatation.
- AR murmur in 2nd aortic area—Valvular lesion.
- AR murmur is increased by hand grip.

Severity

1. Duration of murmur (> 2/3rd of diastole) is directly proportional to the severity.
2. Bisferiens pulse.
3. Hill's sign > 60 mmHg.
4. Apical impulse (down and out).
5. Austin-Flint murmur.
6. Marked peripheral signs.

ECG

LV enlargement (volume overload) – 'q' waves in V_5, V_6.

Chest X-ray

1. Gross cardiomegaly (cor bovinum).
2. In syphilitic AR, there may be calcification of ascending aorta.
3. In bicuspid aortic valve or rheumatic AR, there may be calcification of the aortic valve.

Echocardiogram (Fig. 23.1)

Dilated LV, hyperdynamic ventricle, fluttering anterior mitral leaflet and Doppler detects reflux.

Cardiac Catheterization

Dilated LV, aortic regurgitation and dilated aortic root.

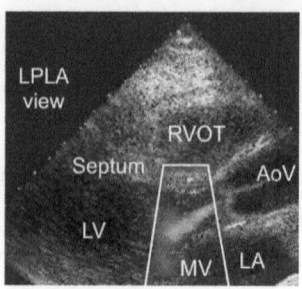

Fig. 23.1: Echo findings in AR

Table 23.1: Differentiating features between acute and chronic AR

Features	Acute AR	Chronic AR
Onset	Early, sudden	Late, insidious
Pulse pressure	Normal	Wide
Systolic pressure	Normal	Increased
Diastolic pressure	Normal	Markedly decreased
LV impulse	Normal	Hyperdynamic
S_1	Soft	Normal
S_3	Common	Uncommon
Peripheral signs	Absent	Present
ECG	Normal LV	LV enlargement
Chest X-ray	Normal LV	Markedly enlarged

Causes of Combined AS and AR

1. Congenital-bicuspid aortic valve.
2. Rheumatic heart disease (usually associated with mitral valve involvement).
3. Systemic lupus erythematosus.
4. Subvalvular AS when complicated by infective endocarditis.

Table 23.2: Differentiating features between rheumatic and syphilitic AR

Features	Rheumatic AR	Syphilitic AR
History	Rheumatic fever	Syphilis
Angina	Less common	Common
Site	Aortic valve	Aortic root
A_2	Normal	Loud tambour-like

Contd...

Contd...

Features	Rheumatic AR	Syphilitic AR
Diastolic murmur-site	Third left sternal border	Second right space (to the right of sternum)
Peripheral signs of AR	Not well-marked	Very well-marked
Other valvular lesions	Common	Never present
VDRL	Negative	Positive

- Syphilitic AR may present as ascending aortic aneurysm.
- Murmur of AR is conducted along the right sternal border in syphilitic AR and AR in Marfan's syndrome.

Management

Medical

- Antifailure measures
- Rheumatic fever prophylaxis
- Infective endocarditis prophylaxis
- Vasodilators like ACE inhibitors.

Acute AR

- Diuretics
- IV nitroprusside
- Surgery.

β-blockers and intra-aortic balloon counter pulsation are contraindicated.

Chronic AR

1. Vasodilators like hydralazine and dihydropyridine calcium channel blockers are useful.
2. Penicillin prophylaxis is essential in syphilitic aortitis.
3. β-blockers are useful in aortic root dilatation with or without AR.
4. The goal is to reduce systolic blood pressure to 140 mmHg.

Surgical

- Early left ventricular systolic dysfunction even in the absence of symptoms is an indication for surgery.
- Valve replacement.
- Echocardiogram must be performed every year and aortic valve replacement is indicated in patients with end-systolic dimension > 55 mm or end-systolic volume > 55 ml/m^2 or ejection fraction < 55% (Rule of 55).

Chapter 24

Tricuspid Stenosis (TS) and Tricuspid Regurgitation (TR)

Tricuspid Stenosis (TS)

- Uncommon valvular lesion
- Usually associated with mitral valve disease
- Tricuspid stenosis (TS) is more common in females.

Causes

- Rheumatic heart disease
- Congenital TS
- Carcinoid syndrome.

When to Entertain the Diagnosis of TS

- When pulmonary congestion disappears in patients with mitral stenosis
- When mitral stenosis findings are masked
- When there is no improvement after mitral stenosis surgery.

Symptoms

- Dyspnea
- Fatigue.

Signs

- Giant 'a' waves in JVP.
- Prominent presystolic pulsations of the liver.
- No palpable P_2 or right ventricular enlargement.
- Occasionally opening snap of tricuspid valve may be heard.
- A diastolic murmur over tricuspid area which increases during inspiration (Carvallo's sign) and reduces during expiration.
- Signs of right heart failure—Ascites, edema, etc.

ECG
- Absence of evidence of right ventricular hypertrophy (RVH) in patients with right-sided failure.

Chest X-ray
- In combined MS and TS, there is prominence of right atrium and superior vena cava (SVC) without much enlargement of pulmonary artery.

Echocardiogram
- Fused and thickened tricuspid valve
- Dilated RA.

Treatment
- Antifailure measures.
- In mild TS, surgery is not ordinarily indicated.
- In moderate to severe TS, definitive surgical treatment is indicated.
- TS is mostly accompanied by TR and in such cases, valve replacement may be indicated.

Tricuspid Regurgitation (TR)
- In the presence of TS, TR is mostly organic
- In the absence of TS, TR is mostly functional.

Causes

Primary
- Rheumatic
- Infective endocarditis (in IV drug addicts)
- Ebstein's anomaly
- Carcinoid syndrome
- Trauma.

Secondary
- Right ventricular dilatation (functional TR as seen in MS or MR with PHT, Eisenmenger's syndrome, PS and primary pulmonary hypertension).
- Right ventricular infarction.
- Dilated cardiomyopathy.
- RV apical pacing.

Symptoms and Signs

- Weakness and fatigue.
- Throbbing pulsations in the neck (raised JVP).
- Cyanosis (right to left shunt through patent foramen ovale).
- Jaundice.
- Massive edema.
- Irregularly irregular pulse (due to AF).
- Jugular venous distension (large, systolic 'CV' wave or 'S' wave).
- A venous systolic thrill and murmur in the neck may be present.
- RV type of apical impulse which is hyperdynamic and thrusting.
- RV S_3.
- P_2 loud when TR is associated with pulmonary hypertension (PHT).
- A high-pitched PSM loudest in 4th intercostal space in the parasternal region augmented during inspiration (Carvallo's sign).
- Systolic hepatic pulsation.
- Positive hepatojugular reflux.
- Ascites.
- Painful congestive hepatomegaly.

Severity

- Murmur is long in severe TR.

ECG

- Nonspecific
- Incomplete RBBB
- 'Q' waves in V_1
- Features of AF.

Chest X-ray

Marked cardiomegaly (prominent RA and RV).

Echocardiogram

- RV dilatation
- Tricuspid valve may be structurally abnormal.

Management

- Isolated TR without PHT is usually well-tolerated.
- Effective correction of mitral valve disease and antifailure measures result in marked improvement.
- Rarely, tricuspid annuloplasty or valve replacement is done.

Chapter 25
Pulmonary Stenosis (PS) and Pulmonary Regurgitation (PR)

Pulmonary Stenosis (PS)

Causes
- Congenital
  - Isolated
  - Associated with VSD (Fallot's tetralogy).
- Carcinoid syndrome
- Rheumatic heart disease.

Pulmonary stenosis is usually of congenital origin. Rheumatic inflammation of the pulmonic valve is very uncommon and is usually associated with involvement of other valves.

Pulmonary Stenosis May Occur at Various Levels
- Supravalvular
- Valvular
- Infundibular
- Subinfundibular.
  - Congenital PS presents as a dome-shaped diaphragm.
  - Supravalvular pulmonary stenosis occurs in congenital rubella syndrome.
  - Concentric hypertrophy of the right ventricle occurs.
  - Marked pulmonary stenosis causes dyspnea and fatigue, and central cyanosis may develop (secondary to right-to-left shunt across foramen ovale).

Pulmonary Stenosis Associated Syndromes
- Maternal rubella
- Noonan syndrome
- Williams syndrome
- Fetal hydantoin syndrome.

- Cutis laxa
- Alagille syndrome
- Leopard syndrome.

Clinical Features

- A raised JVP, with prominent 'a' wave.
- Lower left parasternal heave.
- Systolic thrill felt over pulmonary area.
- S_2 is widely split (mild PS).
- P_2 is soft and delayed, in valvular PS.
- Pulmonary ejection click may be heard, in valvular PS.
- Harsh, loud ejection systolic murmur heard over the pulmonary area, increasing in intensity with inspiration.

ECG

RVH and RBBB.

Chest X-ray

- Right atrial and right ventricular enlargement
- Prominence of the main pulmonary artery.

Complications

- Right ventricular failure
- Infective endocarditis
- Sudden death.

Treatment

Pulmonary balloon valvuloplasty is preferred.
Other corrective surgeries are:
- Pulmonary valvotomy
- Pulmonary valve repair
- Pulmonary valve replacement.

Pulmonary Regurgitation (PR)

Causes

- Idiopathic pulmonary dilatation
- Marfan's syndrome
- Primary pulmonary hypertension
- Infective endocarditis in intravenous (IV) drug addicts

- Trauma
- Secondary.
    a. Eisenmenger's syndrome
    b. Mitral stenosis.

Signs

Graham-Steell murmur—A high-pitched decrescendo diastolic blowing murmur along left sternal border increasing on inspiration.

Table 25.1: Differences between AR and PR

	AR	PR
Signs of wide pulse pressure	Present	Absent
Apex beat	Hyperdynamic	Normal
Relation of murmur to respiration	None	Increases on inspiration
Ventricular enlargement	LVH	RVH

Chapter 26

Pulmonary Hypertension

Pulmonary hypertension is an abnormal elevation in pulmonary artery pressure, may be the result of left heart failure, pulmonary parenchymal or vascular disease, thromboembolism, or a combination of these factors.

Normal pulmonary artery pressures are as follows:
- Systolic pressure — 15–25 mmHg
- Diastolic pressure — 5–10 mmHg
- Mean pressure — 10–15 mmHg

Pulmonary hypertension is present when pulmonary artery systolic pressure is > 30 mmHg, and pulmonary artery mean pressure is > 20 mmHg.

Clinical Classification of Pulmonary Hypertension

Pulmonary arterial hypertension (PAH)
- Idiopathic pulmonary arterial hypertension
- Familial pulmonary arterial hypertension
- Associated pulmonary arterial hypertension
    i. Collagen vascular disease
    ii. Congenital systemic to pulmonary shunts
    iii. Portal hypertension
    iv. HIV infections
    v. Drugs and toxins
    vi. Others—(Glycogen storage disorders, hemoglobinopathies and myeloproliferative disorders).

Pulmonary venous hypertension
- Left-sided atrial or ventricular heart disease
- Left-sided valvular heart disease.

Pulmonary hypertension associated with parenchymal lung disease or chronic hypoxemia
- COPD
- ILD
- Sleep disordered breathing
- Alveolar hypoventilation disorders
- Chronic exposure to high-altitude.

Pulmonary hypertension due to thrombotic or thromboembolic disease
- Thromboembolic obstruction of proximal pulmonary arteries
- Thromboembolic obstruction of distal pulmonary arteries
- Pulmonary embolism.

Pulmonary hypertension due to miscellaneous conditions
- Sarcoidosis
- Pulmonary Langerhans cell histiocytosis
- Lymphangiomatosis.

Compression of pulmonary vessels
- Tumor
- Adenopathy
- Fibrosing mediastinitis.

Clinical Features
- The most common symptom attributable to pulmonary hypertension is exertional dyspnea. Other common symptoms are fatigue, angina pectoris, syncope, near syncope and peripheral edema.
- Physical examination reveals increased jugular venous pressure, loud P_2, a right-sided fourth heart sound, TR murmur, RVH and features of RV failure later.
- Idiopathic pulmonary arterial hypertension (IPAH), formerly referred to as primary pulmonary hypertension, is uncommon. There is a female predominance, with most patients presenting in the fourth and fifth decades.

Functional Assessment of Pulmonary Hypertension
- Class I—No limitation of physical activity.
- Class II—Symptomatic on ordinary physical activity.
- Class III—Marked limitation of physical activity.
- Class IV—Unable to carry out any physical activity—Dyspneic at rest with signs of right heart failure.

Investigations

- Chest X-ray—In severe pulmonary hypertension, enlargement of RV and pulmonary arteries are seen. It may also show evidence of primary lung or cardiac diseases.
- Ventilation-perfusion lung scan—This shows perfusion defects in thromboembolism.
- Pulmonary angiogram—It is indicated when there is suspicion of thromboembolism.
- ECG—P pulmonale, right axis deviation, RV hypertrophy and RBBB (Fig. 26.1).
- The echocardiogram commonly demonstrates RV and right atrial enlargement, a tricuspid regurgitant jet.
- Pulmonary function testing to assess COPD/restrictive disorders.
- Arterial blood gas (ABG)—Low PaO_2 and elevated $PaCO_2$ in case of parenchymal lung disease.
- CT chest—To assess parenchymal and mediastinal lesions.
- Right heart catheterisation—To confirm PAH.
- Lung biopsy—Histologic confirmation of lung pathology.

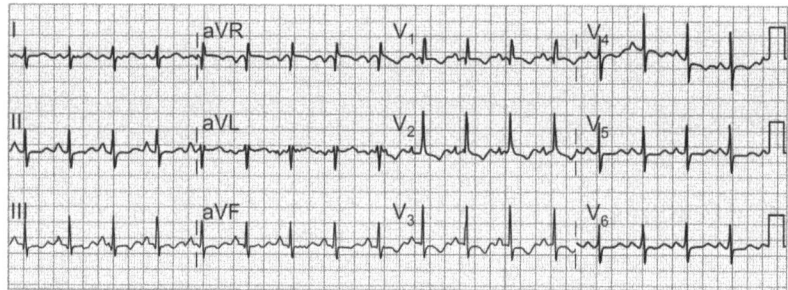

Fig. 26.1: P pulmonale and right ventricular hypertrophy

Management

- Treat the underlying cause.
- Correct hypoxemia with oxygen.
- Diuretics in RV failure.
- Vasodilators in PPH
    - Calcium channel blockers—Nifedipine and diltiazem
    - Angiotensin-converting enzyme inhibitors
    - Epoprostenol and treprostinil
    - Bosentan endothelin receptor antagonist
    - Sildenafil—An oral phosphodiesterase-5 inhibitor.
- Creation of a small ASD by balloon septostomy (allows deoxygenated blood to reach LV improving cardiac output).
- Heart-lung transplant.
- Surgical intervention in thromboembolism.

Chapter 27

Mitral Valve Prolapse (MVP)

Synonyms

- Systolic click-murmur syndrome
- Barlow's syndrome
- Floppy-valve syndrome
- Billowing mitral leaflet syndrome.

Causes

- Myxomatous degeneration of the mitral leaflet tissue.
- A genetically determined collagen disorder—A reduction in the production of type III collagen.
- MVP is a frequent finding in patients with heritable disorders of connective tissue, including Marfan syndrome, osteogenesis imperfecta, and Ehlers-Danlos syndrome. MVP may be associated with thoracic skeletal deformities, such as a high-arched palate and alterations of the chest and thoracic spine, including the so-called straight back syndrome.
- The posterior mitral leaflet is usually more affected than the anterior.
- MVP is seen in 20% of patients with ostium secundum atrial septal defect.

Clinical Features

- MVP is more common in women
- Age incidence—Between 15 and 30 years
- The clinical course is most often benign
- Most patients are asymptomatic and remain so for their entire lives
- Infective endocarditis may occur.

Auscultation

- Midsystolic (nonejection) click due to sudden tensing of elongated chordae tendineae followed by a high-pitched, late systolic crescendo-

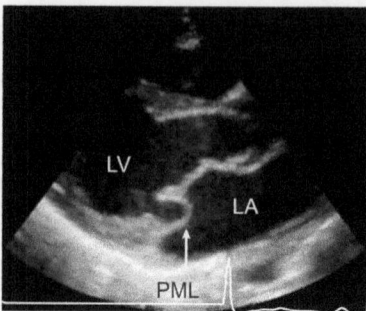

Fig. 27.1: Echo in MVP

decrescendo murmur, which occasionally is "whooping" or "honking" in quality and is heard best at the apex.

Laboratory Examination

- The ECG is normal. Diagnosis is confirmed by echocardiogram (Fig. 27.1).

Treatment

- Mitral valve prolapse.
- Valve repair is rarely indicated.
- Infective endocarditis prophylaxis is indicated only for patients with a prior history of endocarditis.

Chapter 28

Atrial Septal Defect (ASD)

- Most common congenital heart disease
- Asymptomatic until middle age
- ASD is more common in females.

Four Types of ASD

1. Ostium secundum (90%)
2. Ostium primum (5%)
3. Sinus venosus (5%)
4. Coronary sinus type—Very rare.

Ostium primum type

- Associated with Down's syndrome
- With endocardial cushion defects (MR and TR).

Ostium secundum type (Fig. 28.1)

Sporadic or autosomal dominant

Persistent foramen ovale—In about 30% of adults the foramen ovale (PFO) does not close completely, but remains as a small patent foramen ovale. PFO may cause paradoxical embolism. (PFO should be considered as a cause of paradoxical embolism after exclusion of more common causes of stroke).

Syndromes with ASD

1. Holt-Oram syndrome (Ostium secundum ASD)
2. Trisomy 13 (Patau syndrome)
    - ASD, VSD and PDA
3. Trisomy 18 (Edward syndrome)
    - ASD, VSD and PDA

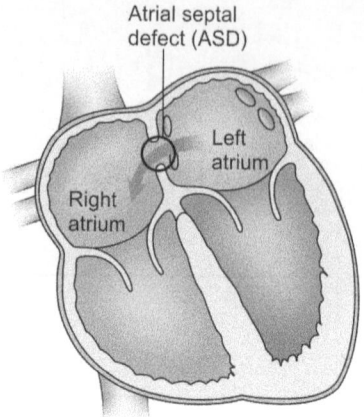

Fig. 28.1: Atrial septal defect

4. Ellis van Crevald syndrome
5. TAR syndrome(thrombocytopenia and absent radius)
6. Trisomy 21 (Down syndrome)
7. Congenital rubella syndrome.

ASD can be associated with

a. MVP
b. Acquired MS (Lutembacher's syndrome).

Sinus venosus type of ASD

Occurs high in the septum near the SVC entrance.
May be associated with partial anomalous pulmonary venous connection.
- AF is common in ASD.
- Infective endocarditis is uncommon in ASD, except in ostium primum type, due to associated MR or TR.

Clinical Features

a. One-third of patients with ASD have a systolic thrill. If thrill is prominent, associated PS should be thought of.
b. Wide, fixed split of S_2 is the characteristic auscultatory finding of ASD
    - S_2 split is narrowed with development of PAH.
    - Split is variable with development of AF.
c. Flow ESM across pulmonary valve.
d. Flow MDM across tricuspid valve.

ECG

a. Ostium secundum: RAD and incomplete RBBB.
b. Ostium primum: LAD with incomplete RBBB.
c. Sinus venosus: Inverted 'P' wave in inferior leads.
d. Junctional rhythm may be present.
e. Rarely ostium primum defects may be associated with complete heart block.

Chest Radiograph

1. Dilated right atrium, right ventricle and pulmonary arteries, with a less prominent aortic knuckle give a characteristic 'jug handle appearance'.
2. The lung fields show increased vascularity.

Echocardiography is done for demonstrating shunts as well as patent foramen ovale.

Treatment

- ASD can close spontaneously upto 2 years of age.
- Surgical closure (ideal age 3–6 years).
- Indication for surgery—Significant shunt with pulmonary to systemic flow > 1.5 : 1.
- A noninvasive procedure is closure of the defect using an umbrella.

Chapter 29

Ventricular Septal Defect (VSD)

Ventricular Septal Defect (VSD) (Fig. 29.1)

Most common congenital heart disease.

Classification

Perimembranous or paramembranous type

- Most common (80%)
- It is also called infracristal, subaortic or conoventricular type.

Muscular type

Muscular type subdivided into 3 types:
  a. Inlet

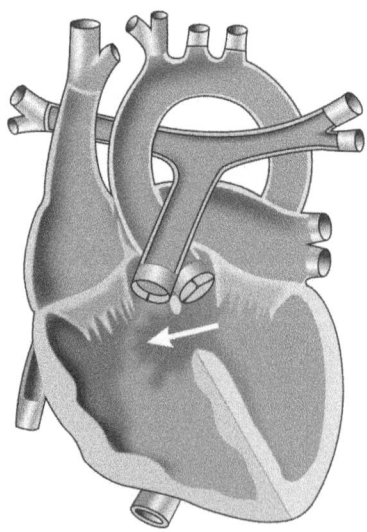

Fig. 29.1: Ventricular septal defect

b. Trabecular (or swiss cheese type)
   c. Outlet. It is also called as supracrispal, subpulmonic, or infundibular.

Syndromes with VSD
- Trisomy's 8,13,18 and 21
- Cri-du-chat syndrome
- Cornelia de Lange syndrome
- Klippel-Feil syndrome
- Velacardio facial syndrome
- Fetal alcohol syndrome
- Apert syndrome
- Conradi-Hunermann syndrome
- Vater association.

Spontaneous closure of the defect may occur in 50% of those having a defect less than 0.5 cm in diameter (in muscular septal defect only) upto 6 years of age.

Mechanism of Closure of Defect
   a. Septal muscle grows around defect.
   b. Prolapsed aortic or tricuspid valve gets adherent to defect with over growth of fibrous tissue.
   c. Infective endocarditis or development of ventricular septal aneurysm may close the defect.

VSD may produce symptoms much earlier in life.

Clinical features
- Grade IV pansystolic murmur over the left sternal border
- Signs of biventricular enlargement.
- Systolic thrill in the left sternal border.
- A mid-diastolic flow murmur may be heard across the mitral valve.
- Occurrence of infective endocarditis is very common specially in small shunts.
- CCF may develop early in large shunts.

Maladie-de-Roger Syndrome
   a. It is a small sized muscular VSD
   b. A prominent thrill
   c. A loud pansystolic murmur
   d. Without any hemodynamic changes
   e. ECG is normal
   f. Spontaneous closure of defect may occur.

ECG

- Evidence of biventricular enlargement
- With or without RBBB
- Occasionally with complete heart block.

Chest X-ray

a. Left ventricular enlargement
b. Pulmonary plethora.

Echocardiogram

- Demonstrates the defect
- Doppler assesses the magnitude of shunting.

Treatment

- Surgical closure is the treatment of choice.
- Ideal age for surgery < 2 years of age.
- Indication for surgery is when pulmonary to systemic blood flow is > 1.5 : 1.

Chapter 30
Patent Ductus Arteriosus (PDA)

The ductus arteriosus is a vessel leading from the bifurcation of the pulmonary artery to the aorta just distal to the left subclavian artery (Fig. 30.1). The ductus arteriosus is a remnant of the distal sixth aortic arch. The ductus arteriosus is normally patent during fetal life. This patency is promoted by continual production of prostaglandin E_2 (PGE_2) by the ductus.

Congenital rubella infection in the first trimester of pregnancy, maternal phenytoin use, premature infants are associated with high incidence of (PDA).

Normally, the ductus closes immediately after birth. A PDA produces a left-to-right shunt. A gradient and shunt from aorta to pulmonary artery persist throughout the cardiac cycle, resulting in a continuous murmur.

Syndromes with PDA
- Maternal rubella syndrome
- Trisomy 18
- Fetal hydantoin syndrome
- Incontinentia pigmenti
- Crouzon's syndrome
- Rubenstein Taybi syndrome
- Conradi-Hunermann syndrome.

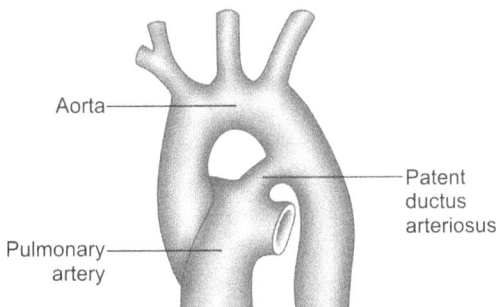

Fig. 30.1: Patent ductus arteriosus

Symptoms

Patients can present at any age. Usually PDA is asymptomatic. The patient may present with lower respiratory tract infections.

Signs

- Brisk arterial pulse
- Wide pulse pressure
- Dynamic LV impulse.

A systolic thrill is present in the left infraclavicular region

A continuous "machinery" murmur is heard over the left second intercostal space at midclavicular line. Synonyms are Gibson murmur, train in the tunnel, windmill murmur. It may be heard in the left 1st intercostal space (Gibson's area) and in the left infraclavicular area.

ECG

- LA, LV and RV enlargement usually seen.

In adults Eisenmenger syndrome develops with pulmonary hypertension, right-to-left shunting, and cyanosis. Severe pulmonary hypertension results in reversal of flow through the ductus; resulting in toes—but not the fingers—become cyanotic and clubbed, a finding termed differential cyanosis and clubbing.

Complications

- Cardiac failure
- Infective endocarditis
- Ductal endarteritis
- Aneurysmal dilatation, calcification and rupture of the ductus.

Treatment of Patent Ductus Arteriosus

Medical

Indomethacin or ibuprofen is usually given within first 2–7 days of life. Indomethacin reduces the PGE levels, favouring the closure of ductus.

Surgical

- Surgical ligation and division remain the standard treatment of PDA.
- Transcatheter closure is also done.

Chapter 31

Tetralogy of Fallot (TOF)

It is the most common cyanotic congenital heart disease in patients who survive infancy.

4 Distinct Anatomic Abnormalities (Fig. 31.1)

- VSD.
- Right ventricular outflow tract obstruction (infundibular pulmonary stenosis).
- Overriding of the aorta.
- Right ventricular hypertrophy.

Embryology

Anterocephalad malalignment of the infundibular septum, resulting in VSD right ventricular outflow tract obstruction and overriding of the aorta.

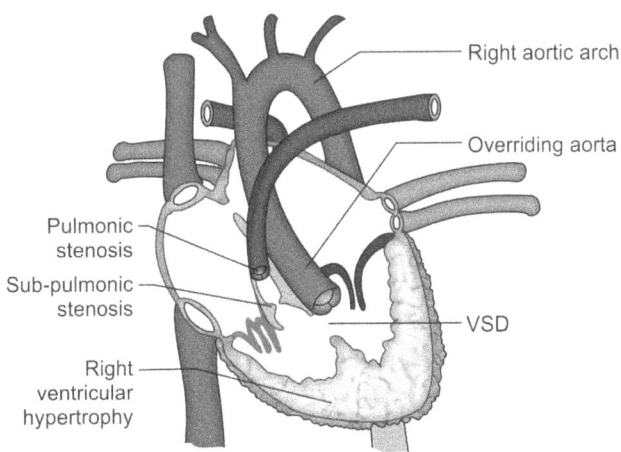

Fig. 31.1: Tetralogy of Fallot

Cyanotic Fallot

When the resistance to pulmonary outflow is greater than the systemic resistance, right to left shunting of blood across the VSD occurs, resulting in central cyanosis.

Acyanotic Fallot

When the resistance to the pulmonary outflow is lower than the systemic resistance, then a predominant left to right shunt occurs across the VSD and cyanosis is absent.

Cyanotic Spells

Initially, in TOF, cyanosis is episodic, occurring during feeding, crying, fever, exercise, etc. when systemic vasodilatation occurs causing an increased right to left shunting across the VSD. A baby born cyanotic is unlikely to have TOF. Cyanosis becomes more prominent after about 5–6 months of life.

Squatting Episodes

A characteristic fashion in which older children with tetralogy of Fallot increase pulmonary blood flow is by squatting. Squatting is a compensatory mechanism, and highly typical of infants with tetralogy of Fallot. Squatting increases peripheral vascular resistance and thus decreases the magnitude of the right-to-left shunt across the VSD.

Associated Cardiac Anomalies

- Patent foramen ovale.
- ASD.
- AR.
- Right-sided aortic arch (it is the most common anomaly, seen in 30% of cases).
- PDA.
- Anomalous origin of the coronary arteries.
- Absence of left pulmonary artery.

Pentology of Fallot—ASD+TOF
Triology of Fallot—PS, RVH and ASD.

Associated Syndromes

- TAR syndrome
- Down syndrome
- DiGeorge syndrome
- CHARGE association
- Velocardiofacial syndrome.

Clinical Features

Symptoms

Dyspnea on exertion, cyanotic spells and squatting episodes.

Signs

- Central cyanosis.
- Clubbing.
- Anemia (due to stunted growth).
- Secondary polycythemia.
- Absence of cardiomegaly, absence of left parasternal heave and absence of palpable P_2.
- Systolic thrill in pulmonary area in 30% of patients.
- A silent precordium is often characteristic.

On Auscultation

- A loud, single S_2 (representing aortic valve closure).
- ESM is best heard over the 3rd and 4th left intercostal spaces conducted to the left shoulder. The intensity and duration of the murmur is inversely proportional to the severity of right ventricular outflow tract (RVOT) obstruction.
- Because of a large ventricular septal defect, VSD murmur is inconspicuous.

ECG

RAD and RVH.

Chest X-ray

1. This shows a normal-sized heart with a characteristic appearance termed as 'Coeur en Sabot' or 'boot-shaped heart' (tilted apex). There is pulmonary oligemia. Boot-shaped heart is due to the prominence of RV and concavity in the region is due to under developed RVOT and main pulmonary artery.
2. Right-sided aortic arch seen in 30% of cases.

Complications

- Marked secondary polycythemia may result in intravascular thrombosis leading to cerebrovascular accident (CVA) and paradoxical emboli.
- Cerebral abscess (common causative organism being *Streptococcus*).
- Infective endocarditis (common causative organism being *Streptococcus*).

Treatment

Medical

Treatment of cyanotic spells by—
- a. Squatting or knee chest position
- b. Nasal O_2
- c. Morphine
- d. β-blockers—propranolol (help to relieve infundibular spasm)
- e. Correct metabolic acidosis.

Surgical

- a. Open heart surgery and total correction is the definitive treatment.
- b. If pulmonary arteries are excessively small, then early definitive correction of TOF is not possible.
- c. A palliative procedure (Blalock-Taussig shunt—Left subclavian to left pulmonary artery) is done till the time when the pulmonary arteries have enlarged sufficiently.
- d. Waterston procedure—Ascending aorta to right pulmonary artery.
- e. Pott's procedure—Descending aorta to left pulmonary artery.

Chapter 32

Eisenmenger's Syndrome

Introduction

- It is the condition in which left to right shunt gets reversed (right to left) with the development of severe pulmonary hypertension, resulting in central cyanosis, clubbing and secondary polycythemia (Fig. 32.1).
- Its incidence is equal in both males and females.
- Since this syndrome is uncommon below 2 years of age, surgical closure of left to right shunt lesions is advocated below 2 years of age.
- Hemoptysis is uncommon, but when it occurs, prognosis is bad, as it is caused by rupture of thin-walled, fragile pulmonary arteries or their small aneurysms.
- Conditions that cause systemic vasodilatation (exercise, fever and hot weather) may exaggerate the shunt from right to left resulting in systemic desaturation and poor tolerance.

EISENMENGER COMPLEX—VSD with reversal of shunt.

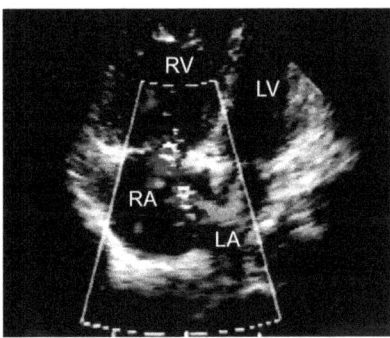

Fig. 32.1: Right to left shunt

Clinical Features

1. Central cyanosis occurs in presence of VSD and ASD.

2. Differential cyanosis involving the lower limbs occurs in the presence of PDA.
3. P_2 is loud and palpable.
4. Prominent left parasternal heave.

Eisenmenger syndrome occurs earlier in life in VSD, a little later in PDA, and very late in adult life in ASD.

- In ASD with reversal — Narrowly fixed split of S_2
- In VSD with reversal — Single S_2 and decreased intensity of murmur
- In PDA with reversal — Closely split S_2

Surgery is not contraindicated in the early phase of Eisenmenger's syndrome.

Death is Caused by

1. Congestive heart failure (CCF)
2. Pulmonary infection
3. Pulmonary infarction
4. Brain abscess
5. Infective endocarditis
6. Severe hemoptysis
7. Ventricular arrhythmias.

Pregnancy must be avoided or terminated with development of Eisenmenger's syndrome.

The only curative treatment of Eisenmenger's syndrome is heart-lung transplantation.

Differential Diagnosis

1. Primary pulmonary hypertension
2. Recurrent pulmonary embolism
3. Idiopathic dilatation of pulmonary artery.

Chapter 33

Coarctation of the Aorta

Coarctation of the aorta is a congenital condition whereby the aorta narrows in the area where the ductus arteriosus inserts. The word "coarctation" means narrowing (Fig. 33.1).

In adults coarctation of the aorta typically consists of discrete diaphragm like ridge that extends into the aortic lumen in the region of the ligamentum arteriosum.

Preductal Coarctation

Diffuse coarctation of the ascending aorta and transverse aortic arch, to the origin of the ductus.

In this condition upper-half of the body is perfused via the systemic circulation, whereas flow to the lower-half of the body comes from the pulmonary artery through a patent ductus arteriosus. This results in differential cyanosis and clubbing, where the lower extremities are cyanotic with clubbing.

Postductal Coarctation

Narrowing of the thoracic aorta immediately distal to the origin of the ductus.

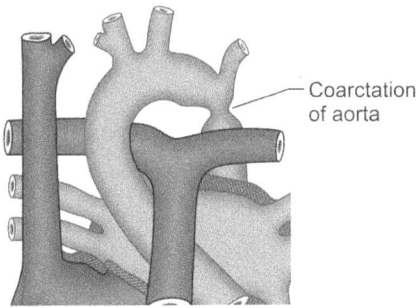

Fig. 33.1: Coarctation of the aorta

Associated Cardiac Anomalies

1. PDA
2. Bicuspid aortic value (80%)
3. VSD.

Coarctation of Aorta Syndromes

1. Turner's syndrome
2. Fetal hydantoin syndrome
3. Crouzon syndrome
4. Increased incidence of berry aneurysm in the circle of Willis.

Clinical Features

Signs and symptoms of cardiac failure does not occur in infancy.

There are usually no symptoms until hypertension produces LVF or cerebral hemorrhage.

1. Systolic arteriolar pressure is higher in the arms than in the legs, but the diastolic pressure is usually similar.
2. Femoral pulses are weak and delayed, in comparison to the radial or brachial pulses.
3. Systolic thrill may be palpable in the suprasternal notch.
4. Left ventricular hypertrophy (LVH) may be present.
5. Prominent suprasternal and neck pulsations are present.
6. Pulsations are present in the back in the suprascapular area and left interscapular area and around the scapula.
7. A systolic ejection click is audible (from a bicuspid aortic valve).
8. A characteristic rough ejection systolic murmur is audible along the left sternal border and in the back.
9. A continuous murmur may be heard over the interscapular or infrascapular areas indicating blood flow through collateral channels.
10. Fundus-Cork screw appearance of retinal arteries.

Coarctation of the abdominal aorta may be associated with renal artery stenosis.

Collateral circulation develops around the coarctation through the intercostals arteries and the branches of the subclavian arteries, enabling blood flow to bypass the obstruction (Fig. 33.2).

Coarctation is a cause of secondary hypertension and should be considered in young patients with elevated BP.

Investigations

ECG

Evidence of LVH seen.

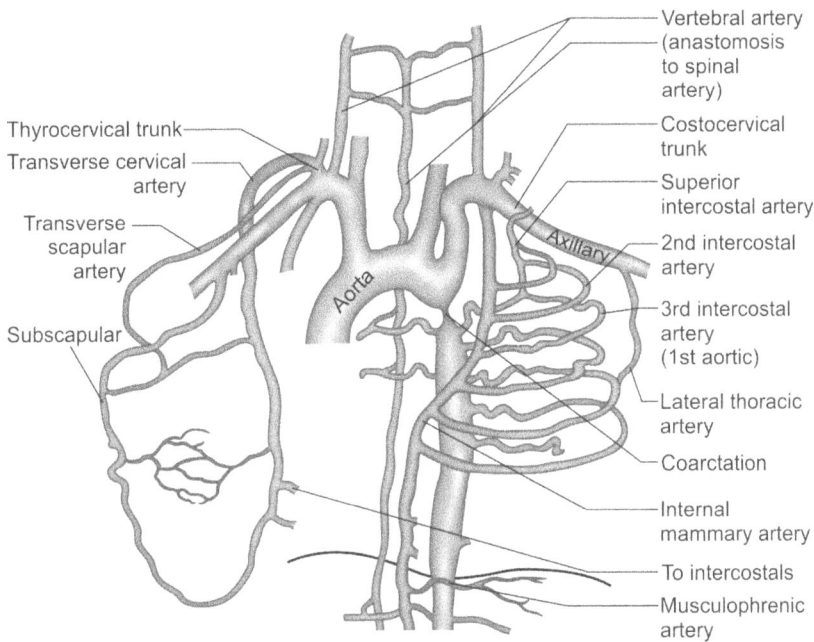

Fig. 33.2: Collateral arculation around the coarctatum

Chest Radiograph

1. Left ventricular hypertrophy (LVH).
2. Notching of the ribs develops along the inferior and posterior aspect of the 3rd–8th ribs bilaterally (Fig. 33.3). It is due to increased flow through the collaterals.
3. Reversed 3 sign (due to pre- and poststenotic aortic dilatation and dilatation of the subclavian artery).

Doppler Echocardiography

It is usually diagnostic and may provide additional evidence for a bicuspid aortic value. Echo/Doppler can also provide estimates of the gradient across the lesion.

Both MRI and CT scan also provide excellent images of the coarctation.

Complications

1. Bacterial endocarditis (at the site of the coarctation, bicuspid aortic valve or associated collateral channels).
2. Aortic dissection and rupture of the proximal ascending aorta may occur sometimes during pregnancy.
3. Rupture of berry aneurysms of the circle of Willis.

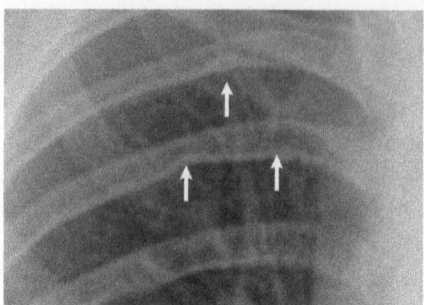

Fig. 33.3: Rib notching

Treatment

Patient with a demonstrated gradient of >20 mm of mercury should be considered for intervention specially if there is evidence of collateral blood results.

Resection of the coarctation site has a surgical mortality rate of 1–4% and includes risk of spinal cord injury.

Treatment of Choice

1. Percutaneous catheter balloon with stent dilatation is now a viable option for many patients.
2. Surgical resection with end-to-end anastamosis. About 25% of patients surgically corrected continue to be hypertensive (secondary hypertension) due to permanent changes in the renin angiotensin system and needs follow up treatment with drugs.

Chapter 34

Other Congenital Heart Diseases

Malpositions of the Heart

Positional anomalies refer to conditions in which the cardiac apex is—
- In the right side of the chest (dextrocardia).
- At the midline (mesocardia).
- There is a normal location of the heart in the left side of the chest but abnormal position of the viscera (isolated levocardia).

Dextrocardia

Dextrocardia with situs inversus (situs inversus totalis) (Fig. 34.1)

Dextrocardia, with situs inversus is the relatively common condition that is usually an incidental finding on chest X-ray (air in fundus of stomach on the right side) or physical examination and is generally benign. About 90% of patients with this condition have hearts that are otherwise normal.

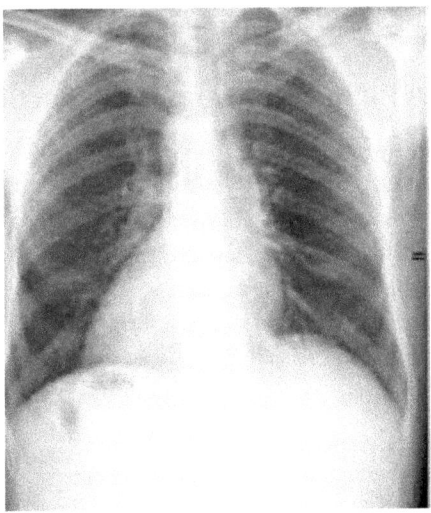

Fig. 34.1: Situs inversus totalis

The ECG Shows Negative P-wave in Standard Lead I (Fig. 34.2)

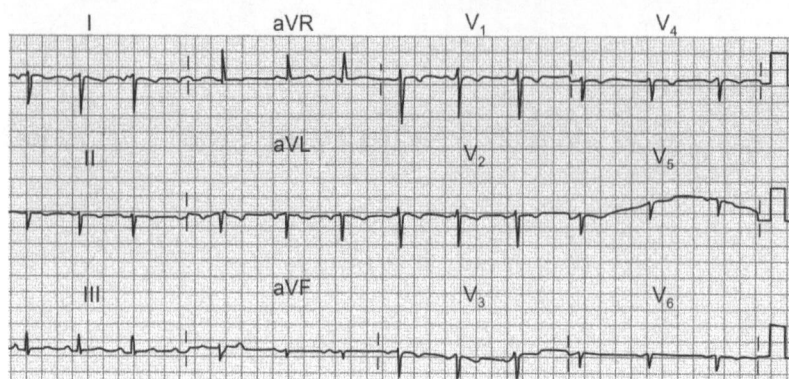

Fig. 34.2: Negative P in lead I

Isolated Dextrocardia

Patients with isolated dextrocardia without situs inversus almost invariably have additional cardiac malformations, the most common being—
 i. Corrected transposition of the great vessels
 ii. Pulmonic stenosis
 iii. Ventricular septal defect
 iv. Atrial septal defect.

Anomalous Pulmonary Venous Connection

- Pulmonary veins drain into a site other than the left atrium.
- 2 types—Partial anomalous pulmonary venous connection (PAPVC) and total anomalous pulmonary venous connection (TAPVC).

Total Anomalous Pulmonary Venous Connection (TAPVC)

- Almost all patients are cyanotic.
- Continuous murmur along left sternal border due to flow through anomalous pulmonary venous channels.
- P_2 is accentuated with development of pulmonary hypertension (PHT) and the murmur becomes less marked.
- TAPVC, with large left to right shunt resembles ostium secundum ASD (except for cyanosis).
- Chest X-ray—Snowman or figure of eight appearance.

Partial Anomalous Pulmonary Venous Connection (PAPVC)

- One or more (but not all) of the pulmonary veins are connected to the right atrium.

- The right lung is involved 10 times more frequently.
- An ASD generally accompanies PAPVC is usually of the sinus venosus type.
- The physical findings in patient with PAPVC are similar to those of an ASD.

Treatment of TAPVC and PAPVC is total surgical correction.

Ebstein's Anomaly (Fig. 34.3)

- Ebstein's anomaly is a congenital malformation involving the tricuspid valve.
- Low set tricuspid valve apparatus causes a portion of the right to be "atrialised".
- The right atrium is dilated, since it consists of a normal right atrium plus the atrialised portion of the right ventricle.
- Associated cardiac abnormalities—ASD, VSD and mitral valve prolapse.
- Many patients are asymptomatic until the third or fourth decade.
- They typically develop cyanosis, usually with exertion (intermittent cyanosis).
- The S_1 is typically loud and widely split.
- The S_2 is widely split.
- Multiple systolic clicks.
- Right-sided S_3 or S_4 may be heard.
- Multiplicity of heart sounds—6 sounds-split S_1, split S_2, S_3, S_4.
- A murmur of tricuspid regurgitation and tricuspid stenosis are heard.
- Chest X-ray—A globular heart (enlarged right atrium).
- ECG—Himalayan 'P' waves (giant, peaked 'P' waves), prolonged PR interval and RBBB.
- Treatment—Surgical correction.

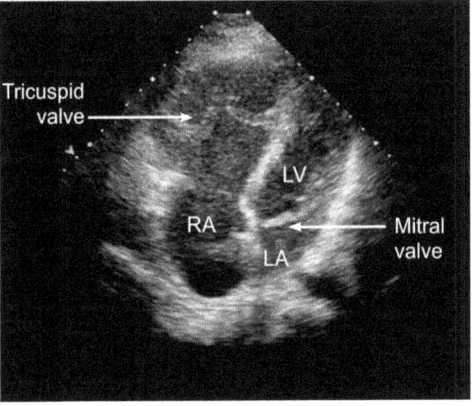

Fig. 34.3: Ebstein's anomaly

Complete Transposition of the Great Vessels (D-transposition)

- D-transposition of the great arteries is the most common cause of cyanotic congenital heart disease in the neonate, after TOF.
- It is a potentially lethal condition.
- In complete transposition of the great vessels, the aorta arises from the right ventricle and pulmonary artery originates from the left ventricle.
- Normal S_1 and single loud S_2.
- ECG— It shows evidence of right ventricular hypertrophy.
- Chest X-ray— "Egg-on-a-stalk" appearance.
- Definitive treatment is surgical ("arterial switch" operation).

Congenitally Corrected Transposition of the Great Vessels

There is both atrioventricular discordance (the atria are connected to the opposite ventricles) and ventriculoarterial discordance (the ventricles are connected to the opposite great vessels).

It is also known as L-transposition of the great vessels.

Truncus Arteriosus

- A single common vessel forms the outflow tract for both ventricles and subsequently gives rise to the systemic, pulmonary and coronary arterial circulation.
- It is always associated with a large supracristal VSD.
- DiGeorge syndrome is associated with truncus arteriosus.

Tricuspid Atresia

- The tricuspid valve is absent.
- The floor of the right atrium is intact.
- Systemic venous blood flows from the right atrium, through an interatrial septum, to the left atrium.
- There is nearly always presence of a ventricular septal defect.
- Central cyanosis (since birth).
- ECG—Left axis deviation.
- Chest X-ray—Heart shows the 'tilted' appearance.
- Pulmonary oligemia is seen.
- Treatment—Surgical correction.

Coronary Arteriovenous Fistula

- It is a communication between a coronary artery and a cardiac chamber
- The fistula most commonly arises from the right coronary artery

- Usually drains into the right ventricle, right atrium or coronarysinus
- It results in a left-to-right shunt
- Patients are generally asymptomatic
- A continuous murmur is heard at the lower sternal border.

Cor Triatriatum (or Triatrial Heart)

It is a congenital heart defect where the left atriumor right atrium is subdivided by a thin membrane, resulting in 3 atrial chambers (hence the name).

Ellis Van Creveld Syndrome

Atrioventricular septal defects (AVSD) including ASD can occur.

Chapter 35

Heart Failure (HF)

Cardiac failure occurs when the heart fails to maintain sufficient circulation to provide adequate tissue oxygenation in the presence of normal filling pressures.

Preload

Preload is the left ventricular end-diastolic pressure and it depends on left ventricular compliance and venous return.

Afterload

Afterload is the left ventricular systolic wall tension that develops during ventricular systole.

Classification of Cardiac Failure

High output and low output failure.

High Output Failure

The normal heart fails to maintain an increased output, in the face of grossly elevated requirements, as in anemia, hyperthyroidism, Paget's disease, A-V malformation and beriberi in pregnancy.

Low Output Failure

The heart fails to generate adequate output, or can only do so with high filling pressures, as in—
  i. Intrinsic heart muscle disease (cardiomyopathy, CAD, myocarditis and Chagas' disease).
  ii. Chronic excessive afterload (aortic stenosis and hypertension).
  iii. Chronic excessive preload (mitral regurgitation).
  iv. Negative inotropic drugs (antiarrhythmic agents).

v. Restricted filling (constrictive pericarditis or tamponade and restrictive cardiomyopathy).
vi. Extreme bradycardia (β-blockers and complete heart block).

Right and Left-sided Heart Failure and Congestive Cardiac Failure

Right-sided Heart Failure

This causes peripheral edema, congestive tender hepatomegaly, raised JVP and hypotension.

Left-sided Heart Failure

Most prominent sign is the presence of pulmonary edema characterized by cyanosis, tachypnea, tachycardia, pink frothy sputum, third heart sound, pulsus alternans and cardiomegaly. Pulmonary crackles (rales or crepitations) result from the transudation of fluid from the intravascular space into the alveoli. In patients with pulmonary edema, rales may be heard widely over both lung fields and may be accompanied by expiratory wheezing (cardiac asthma).

Congestive Cardiac Failure

Patient has features of both right and left-sided heart failure.

Forward and Backward Heart Failure

Forward Heart Failure

This results from an inadequate discharge of blood into the arterial system leading to poor tissue perfusion.

Backward Heart Failure

This results from the failure of one or the other ventricle to fill normally.

Systolic and Diastolic Failure

Systolic Failure

It occurs when there is inadequate cardiac output.

Diastolic Failure

It occurs when there is increased resistance to ventricular inflow and reduced ventricular diastolic capacity.

Table 35.1: New York Heart Association Classification—Classifies dyspnea, angina, fatigue and palpitation to Class I to Class IV based on the functional capacity of the heart

Functional capacity	Objective assessment
Class I	Patients with cardiac disease but without resulting limitation of physical activity
Class II	Patients with cardiac disease resulting in slight limitation of physical activity
Class III	Patients with cardiac disease resulting in marked limitation of physical activity
Class IV	Patients with cardiac disease resulting in inability to carry on any physical activity without discomfort. Symptoms of heart failure or the anginal syndrome may be present even at rest

Left Ventricular Remodeling

Ventricular remodeling refers to the changes in LV mass, volume, and shape and the composition of the heart that occur after cardiac injury and/or abnormal hemodynamic loading conditions.

Clinical Manifestations

Symptoms

The cardinal symptoms of heart failure are fatigue and exertional dyspnea (Table 35.1).

Orthopnea

Orthopnea, which is defined as dyspnea occurring in the recumbent position, is usually a later manifestation of heart failure than is exertional dyspnea. Orthopnea may be relieved by sitting upright at the side of the bed with the legs in a dependent position.

Paroxysmal Nocturnal Dyspnea (PND)

This term refers to acute episodes of severe shortness of breath and coughing that generally occur at night and awaken the patient from sleep, usually 1–3 hours after the patient retires. PND may be manifest by coughing or wheezing.

Cardiac asthma is closely related to PND, is characterized by wheezing secondary to bronchospasm.

Cheyne-Stokes Respiration

It is also referred to as periodic respiration or cyclic respiration, Cheyne-Stokes respiration is present in 40% of patients with advanced heart failure and usually is associated with low cardiac output. There is hyperventilation, followed by period of apnea.

Other Symptoms
- Gastrointestinal symptoms—Anorexia, nausea, early satiety and right-upper-quadrant pain.
- Cerebral symptoms—Confusion, disorientation, sleep and mood disturbances.
- Nocturia is common in heart failure and may contribute to insomnia.

Cardiac Examination
A third heart sound (S_3) is audible at the apex. An S_3 (or protodiastolic gallop) is present in patients with volume overload and it signifies severe heart failure. A fourth heart sound (S_4) is not a specific indicator of heart failure but is usually present in patients with diastolic dysfunction. The murmurs of mitral and tricuspid regurgitation are frequently present in patients with advanced heart failure.

Abdomen and Extremities
Hepatomegaly is an important sign in patients with HF. The enlarged liver is tender and may pulsate during systole if tricuspid regurgitation is present. Ascites is a late sign. Jaundice, also a late finding in HF, results from cardiac cirrhosis.

Peripheral edema is a cardinal manifestation of HF, is usually symmetric and dependent in HF and occurs predominantly in the ankles and the pretibial region in ambulatory patients. In bedridden patients, edema may be found in the sacral area (presacral edema) and the scrotum. Long-standing edema may be associated with indurated and pigmented skin.

Cardiac Cachexia
With severe chronic heart failure, there may be marked weight loss and cachexia. Cachexia augurs a poor overall prognosis.

Framingham Criteria for Diagnosis of Congestive Cardiac Failure (CCF)
Major criteria
- Paroxysmal nocturnal dyspnea
- Neck vein distension
- Bibasilar crackles in the lung fields
- Cardiomegaly
- Acute pulmonary edema
- Third heart sound—Gallop rhythm

- Increased venous pressure (>16 cmH$_2$O)
- Positive hepatojugular reflex.

Minor criteria
- Extremity edema
- Nocturnal cough
- Dyspnea on exertion
- Hepatomegaly
- Pleural effusion
- Tachycardia (>120 bpm)
- Decreased vital capacity by 1/3rd.

Major/minor criteria
- 5 days treatment causing weight loss > 4.5 kg
- For diagnosis: 1 major + 2 minor criteria.

Investigations

Routine laboratory testing

Complete blood count, a panel of electrolytes, blood urea nitrogen, serum creatinine, hepatic enzymes and a urinalysis. Selected patients should have assessment for diabetes mellitus (fasting plasma glucose), dyslipidemia (fasting lipid panel) and thyroid abnormalities (thyroid-stimulating hormone level).

Electrocardiogram (ECG)

A routine 12-lead ECG is recommended. The major importance of the ECG is to assess cardiac rhythm and determine the presence of LV hypertrophy or a prior MI (presence or absence of Q waves). A normal ECG virtually excludes LV systolic dysfunction.

Chest X-ray
- Prominent upper lobe veins pulmonary capillary wedge pressure (PCWP = 15 mmHg).
- Kerley B lines (engorged peripheral lymphatics seen in the lower zones. (PCWP = 20 mmHg).
- Fluid in the fissures or interlobar effusion, known as 'phantom tumor' as it disappears with the treatment of left-sided failure.
- Bat's wing or inverted moustache appearance—Features of pulmonary edema (PCWP= 25 mmHg).
- Pleural effusion may be bilateral and symmetrical, but if unilateral, is usually right-sided.
- Cardiomegaly.

Two-dimensional (2-D) echocardiogram/doppler

For assessment of LV function. The most useful index of LV function is the ejection fraction (EF) (stroke volume divided by end-diastolic volume). When the EF is normal (>50%), systolic function is usually adequate, and when the EF is significantly depressed (<30–40%), contractility is usually depressed.

Biomarkers

B-type natriuretic peptide (BNP) and N-terminal pro-BNP, which are released from the failing heart, are relatively sensitive markers for the presence of heart failure with depressed EF. Other biomarkers, such as troponin T and I, C-reactive protein, tumor necrosis factor (TNF) receptors and uric acid, may be elevated in heart failure and provide important prognostic information.

Management of Acute Heart Failure (Acute Pulmonary Edema)

1. Sitting position with back rest.
2. Oxygen inhalation.
3. If oxygenation is inadequate—Mechanical ventilation.
4. Strict bed rest, pain control and anxiety relief.
5. Treatment of precipitating disorders— Hypertension (HTN), acute myocardial infarction (MI), CAD, volume overload and arrhythmias.
6. Morphine sulfate 5 mg IV. It may be repeated if necessary.
7. Frusemide 40–80 mg IV and can be repeated to a maximum dose of 200 mg.
8. Nitroglycerin—As IV infusion in an initial dose of 20 mcg/minute.
9. IV Nitroprusside—In hypertensive emergencies.
10. Inotropic agents like dopamine, dobutamine and milrinone in case of hypotension or shock.
11. Recombinant BNP (nesiritide) IV bolus followed by IV infusion.
12. Correction of electrolyte imbalance and acidosis.

Nonpharmacologic Measures

Physical rest

In acute phase, absolute bed rest is advised. Early ambulation is advocated to avoid deep vein thrombosis.

Diet

- Dietary restriction of sodium (2–3 gm daily) is recommended in all patients with heart failure.

- Fluid restriction.
- Caloric supplementation is recommended for patients with advanced heart failure and cardiac cachexia.

Drugs for Heart Failure

Diuretics

Diuretics are the only pharmacologic agents that can adequately control fluid retention in advanced heart failure, and they restore and maintain normal volume status in patients with congestive symptoms (dyspnea, orthopnea and edema) or signs of elevated filling pressures (rales, jugular venous distension and peripheral edema). Furosemide, torsemide and bumetanide (loop diuretics) and potassium-sparing diuretics such as spironolactone are used.

Angiotensin Converting Enzyme (ACE) Inhibitors

ACE inhibitors should be used in symptomatic and asymptomatic patients with a depressed EF (<40%). ACE inhibitors stabilize LV remodeling, improve symptoms, reduce hospitalization, and prolong life. ACE inhibitors should be initiated in low doses, followed by gradual increments if the lower doses have been well-tolerated. Captopril, enalapril, lisinopril and ramipril are the ACE inhibitors used.

Angiotensin II Receptor Blockers (ARBs)

It should be used in symptomatic and asymptomatic patients with an EF <40% who are intolerant to ACE inhibitors. Losartan, telmisartan, olmesartan, candesartan, irbesartan and valsartan are the drugs used.

Adrenergic Receptor Blockers

β-blocker therapy represents a major advance in the treatment of patients with a depressed EF. When given in concert with ACE inhibitors, β-blockers reverse the process of LV remodeling, improve patient symptoms, prevent hospitalization and prolong life. Therefore, β-blockers are indicated for patients with symptomatic or asymptomatic HF and a depressed EF <40%, e.g. carvedilol, bisoprolol and metoprolol.

Aldosterone Antagonists

Spironolactone or eplerenone have beneficial effects. It is recommended for patients with New York Heart Association (NYHA) class IV or class III HF who have a depressed EF (<35%).

Digoxin

1. It is recommended for patients with symptomatic LV systolic dysfunction who have concomitant atrial fibrillation.
2. Therapy with digoxin is commonly initiated and maintained at a dose of 0.125–0.25 mg daily.
3. The serum digoxin level should be <1 ng/mL.

Anticoagulation and Antiplatelet Therapy

1. Treatment with warfarin [(INR) 2–3] is recommended for patients with heart failure and chronic or paroxysmal atrial fibrillation or with a history of systemic or pulmonary emboli, including stroke or transient ischemic attack.
2. Aspirin is recommended in heart failure patients with ischemic heart disease for the prevention of MI and death. However, lower doses of aspirin (75 or 81 mg) may be preferable.

Management of Cardiac Arrhythmias

1. Amiodarone is the preferred drug for restoring and maintaining sinus rhythm.
2. Biventricular pacing, also termed cardiac resynchronization therapy.
3. Implantable cardiac defibrillators.

Cardiac Transplantation

For advanced heart failure is being done nowadays.

Chapter 36

Pulmonary Thromboembolism (Acute Cor Pulmonale)

Pulmonary thromboembolism is due to detached thrombi from deep veins of leg (80%); of pelvic veins (10%); or other veins and right-sided cardiac chambers (5%) and very rare causes air, fat, tumor cells, placental bits, amniotic fluid and parasites—Schistosomes (5%).

Ninety percent of deaths occur within the first hour.

Risk Factors for Deep Vein Thrombosis

- Deficiency of antithrombin III, protein C and protein S.
- Presence of lupus anticoagulant.
- Homocystinuria.
- Surgical procedures of more than 30 minutes duration.
- Prolonged bed rest following medical illness or surgery or fractures involving lower limbs.
- Chronic deep venous insufficiency.
- Malignancy predisposes to deep vein thrombosis (DVT).
- Obesity.
- Oral contraceptives.
- Estrogen therapy.
- Congestive heart failure.
- Chronic lung disease.
- Hypertension.
- Diabetes mellitus.
- Inflammatory bowel disorders.
- Varicose veins.
- Pregnancy/postpartum.
- Long distance air travel.
- Cerebrovascular disorder.
- Indwelling central venous catheters.
- Cigaret smoking.
- Paroxysmal nocturnal hemoglobinuria.

Pulmonary Thromboembolism (Acute Cor Pulmonale) 141

1. Deep vein thrombosis usually develops in the region of a venous valve.
2. Large extensive thrombi can develop within a few minutes.
3. Larger leg veins (popliteal and above) are the common source of pulmonary emboli.
4. Pain, warmth and swelling of legs denote deep vein thrombosis.

Clinical Features

The classical manifestations of pulmonary thromboembolism are:
- Unexplained dyspnea
- Tachycardia
- Central chest pain or pleurisy
- Hemoptysis
- In patients with a predisposing condition like DVT.

The clinical signs and the results of investigations vary depending on the size of pulmonary vessels involved—Large (massive), medium (segmental), or pulmonary microvasculature.
- Shock
- Central cyanosis
- Raised JVP
- Dyspnea
- Tachycardia
- Hypotension
- Loud and widely split P_2
- Signs of RV failure
- Gallop rhythm
- Pleural rub and crackles
- Pleural effusion
- Urine output—Reduced
- Low-grade fever.

Investigations

- Doppler venography is the gold-standard technique for diagnosing DVT.
- CT venography—It allows visualization of veins in the abdomen, pelvis and lower extremities.
- MRI venography—It is noninvasive for the diagnosis of acute symptomatic proximal DVT.
- PE specific testing:
  1. Contrast enhanced spiral chest CT
  2. Multidetector CT
  3. V/Q (ventilation perfusion) scanning—Areas of defective perfusion

4. MR angiography
5. Pulmonary angiography—Gold-standard for diagnosing PE.

ECG (Fig. 36.1)

- $S_1Q_3T_3$—S in lead I, Q in lead III and inverted T in lead III strain
- Right axis deviation
- Atrial fibrillation (AF)
- Right bundle-branch block
- Right ventricular hypertrophy (RVH).

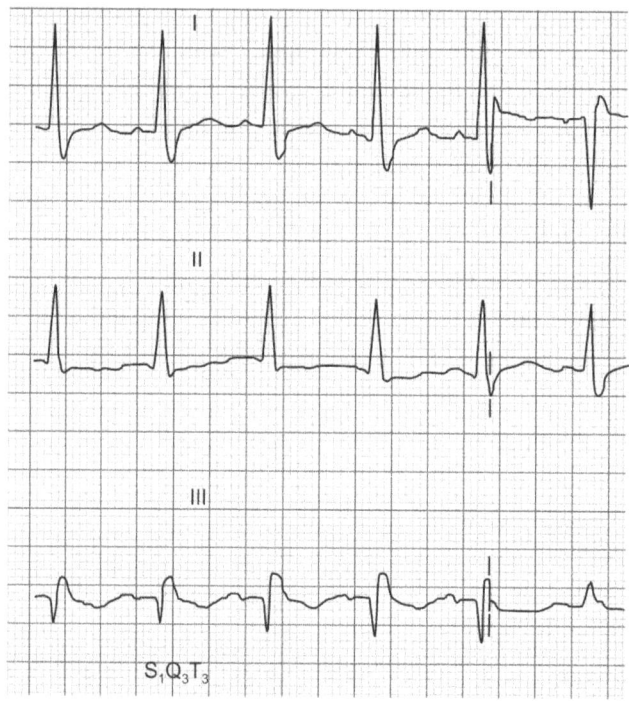

Fig. 36.1: $S_1Q_3T_3$

Chest X-ray

- Hilar prominence
- Raised hemidiaphragm
- Prominent pulmonary trunk and RV
- Oligemic lung fields
- Wedge-shaped or linear opacities
- Pleural effusion.

Blood Gas Analysis
- Reduced PaO_2
- Reduced $PaCO_2$.

Management
1. Administer oxygen (upto 100%).
2. Morphine 10 mg IV if patient is distressed.
3. Heparin—10,000 units IV bolus followed by continuous intravenous—1000 units/hour. Subcutaneous low molecular weight heparin is equally effective. Heparin therapy is given for 10 days.
4. Thrombolytic therapy with streptokinase or urokinase is useful in massive embolism.
5. Pulmonary embolectomy.
6. Venous interruption—Transvenous placement of filter in the inferior vena cava to protect against emboli greater than 2 mm in diameter.
7. Oral anticoagulants like warfarin for 3 months after heparin therapy.

Chapter 37

Cor Pulmonale (Pulmonary Heart Disease)

Definition

Cor pulmonale is defined as dilation and hypertrophy of the right ventricle, with or without failure, secondary to diseases of the pulmonary vasculature, lung parenchyma, thoracic cage abnormalities or ventilation-perfusion defects (Fig. 37.1).

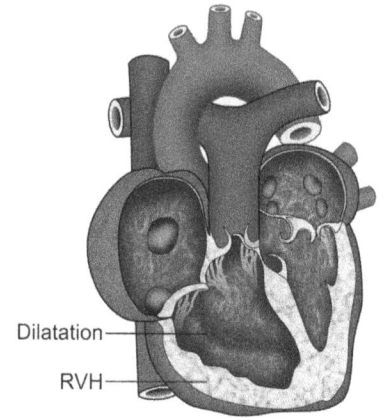

Fig. 37.1: Cor pulmonale

Etiology of Chronic Cor Pulmonale (Table 37.1)

Table 37.1: Etiology of chronic cor pulmonale

Chronic obstructive pulmonary disease
Cystic fibrosis
Chronic hypoventilation • Obesity • Neuromuscular disease • Chest wall dysfunction—Kyphoscoliosis

Contd...

Contd...

High altitude
Pulmonary embolism
Pulmonary arterial hypertension
Pulmonary veno-occlusive disease
Schistosomiasis
Metastatic carcinoma
Sleep apnea syndrome
Bronchiectasis
Pneumoconiosis
Sarcoidosis
Interstitial lung disease

Pulmonary hypertension leads to RV dilation and RV hypertrophy eventually causing the RV to fail.

Clinical Manifestations

Symptoms

- Exertional dyspnea
- Exertional syncope
- Abdominal pain and ascites
- Lower-extremity edema.

Signs

- Tachypnea.
- Elevated jugular venous pressures.
- Hepatomegaly.
- Lower-extremity edema.
- Prominent 'v' waves in JVP due to tricuspid regurgitation.
- Left parasternal heave.
- Epigastric pulsations.
- The increase in intensity of holosystolic murmur of tricuspid regurgitation (TR) with inspiration (Carvallo's sign).
- Cyanosis is a late finding in cor pulmonale.

Diagnosis

ECG

- P pulmonale

- Right axis deviation
- RV hypertrophy.

Chest X-ray

Enlargement of main pulmonary artery, hilar vessels and descending right pulmonary artery.

Spirometry

Obstructive and/or restrictive defects indicative of parenchymal lung diseases.

Arterial blood gases

Demonstrate hypoxemia and/or hypercapnia.

High-resolution computed tomography (HRCT) scans of the chest

It is useful in diagnosing acute thromboembolic disease and interstitial lung disease.

Ventilation-perfusion lung scanning

For diagnosing chronic thromboembolic disease.

Echocardiography

Measures RV thickness and chamber dimensions as well as the anatomy of the pulmonary and tricuspid valves.

Doppler echocardiography can be used to assess pulmonary artery pressures.

Right-heart catheterization is useful for confirming the diagnosis of pulmonary hypertension and for excluding elevated left-heart pressures (measured as the PCWP) as a cause for right-heart failure.

BNP and N-terminal BNP levels are elevated in patients with cor pulmonale secondary to RV stretch and may be dramatically elevated in acute pulmonary embolism.

Treatment

The primary treatment goal of cor pulmonale is to target the underlying pulmonary disease.

General principles of treatment

- Decreasing work of breathing by noninvasive mechanical ventilation and bronchodilation.
- Treating any underlying infection.
- Adequate oxygenation (oxygen saturation 90–92%).

- Correcting respiratory acidosis.
- Blood transfusion in anemia.
- Phlebotomy may be considered in extreme cases of polycythemia.
- Diuretics are effective in RV failure.
- Pulmonary vasodilators are used when isolated pulmonary arterial hypertension is present.

Chapter 38

Systemic Hypertension

Hypertension is defined as a systolic blood pressure (SBP) of 140 mmHg or more, or a diastolic blood pressure (DBP) of 90 mmHg or more, or taking antihypertensive medication.

Based on recommendations of the Seventh Report of the Joint National Committee on Prevention, Detection, Evaluation, and Treatment of High Blood Pressure (JNC7), the classification of blood pressure for adults aged 18 years or older is as follows:
- Normal: Systolic lower than 120 mmHg, diastolic lower than 80 mmHg
- Prehypertension: Systolic 120–39 mmHg, diastolic 80–89 mmHg
- Stage 1: Systolic 140–59 mmHg, diastolic 90–99 mmHg
- Stage 2: Systolic 160 mmHg or greater, diastolic 100 mmHg or greater.

The classification above is based on the average of 2 or more readings taken at each of 2 or more visits after initial screening.

Prehypertension, a new category designated in the JNC7 report, emphasizes that patients with prehypertension are at risk for progression to hypertension and that lifestyle modifications are important preventive strategies.

JNC8 Guidelines Brought the Following Changes

Adjust age-based criteria to define hypertension
- Patients 18–60 years: < 140/90 mmHg
- Patients > 60 years < 150/90 mmHg.

Hypertensive Crises

Hypertensive crises, are defined as a blood pressure of more than 180/120 mmHg classified into hypertensive emergencies and urgencies.

Hypertensive emergencies are characterized by evidence of target organ damage.

Acute end-organ damage in the setting of a hypertensive emergency may include the following:
- Neurologic: Hypertensive encephalopathy, cerebral vascular accident/cerebral infarction, subarachnoid hemorrhage and intracranial hemorrhage.
- Cardiovascular: Myocardial ischemia/infarction, acute left ventricular dysfunction, acute pulmonary edema, aortic dissection and unstable angina pectoris.
- Other: Acute renal failure/insufficiency, retinopathy, eclampsia and microangiopathic hemolytic anemia.

Hypertensive urgencies are those situations without progressive target organ damage.

Etiology

Primary or essential hypertension

It may develop as a result of environmental or genetic causes, excess dietary salt intake and increased adrenergic tone; primary or essential hypertension accounts for 90–95% of adult cases.

Secondary hypertension

It has multiple etiologies, including renal, vascular and endocrine causes. Secondary hypertension accounts for 2–10% of cases.

Causes of secondary hypertension

1. Renal causes of hypertension include the renal parenchymal diseases and renal vascular diseases. Causes include—
   - Polycystic kidney disease
   - Chronic kidney disease
   - Obstructive uropathy
   - Renin-producing tumor
   - Liddle syndrome
   - Renovascular hypertension.
2. Vascular causes include the followings:
   - Coarctation of aorta
   - Vasculitis
   - Collagen vascular disease.
3. Endocrine causes include the followings:
   - Primary hyperaldosteronism
   - Cushing syndrome
   - Pheochromocytoma
   - Congenital adrenal hyperplasia

- Hyperthyroidism and hypothyroidism
        - Hyperparathyroidism
        - Acromegaly.
4. Neurogenic causes
    - Brain tumor
    - Bulbar poliomyelitis
    - Intracranial hypertension
    - Guillain-Barré syndrome.
5. Drugs and toxins
    - Alcohol
    - Cocaine
    - Cyclosporine and tacrolimus
    - Nonsteroidal anti-inflammatory drugs (NSAIDs)
    - Erythropoietin
    - Adrenergic medications
    - Decongestants containing ephedrine
    - Herbal remedies containing licorice
    - Nicotine
    - Estrogen use.
6. Other causes:
    - Hypercalcemia
    - Obstructive sleep apnea
    - Pregnancy-induced hypertension.

Clinical Presentation (Table 38.1)

Table 38.1: Approach to a patient with hypertension

Approach to a patient with hypertension
Duration of hypertension
Previous therapies
Family history of hypertension and cardiovascular disease
Dietary and psychosocial history
Other risk factors: Weight change, dyslipidemia, smoking, diabetes and physical inactivity
Evidence of secondary hypertension: History of renal disease, muscle weakness, spells of sweating, palpitations, tremor, erratic sleep, snoring, daytime somnolence, and symptoms of hypo- or hyperthyroidism
Evidence of target organ damage: History of transient ischemic attack (TIA), stroke, transient blindness, angina, myocardial infarction and congestive heart failure

Symptoms

Most patients with hypertension have no specific symptoms referable to their blood pressure elevation. Although popularly considered a symptom of elevated arterial pressure; headache generally occurs only in patients with severe hypertension. Characteristically, a "hypertensive headache" occurs in the morning and is localized to the occipital region. Other nonspecific symptoms that may be related to elevated blood pressure include dizziness, palpitations, easy fatigability and impotence.

Physical Examination

Body habitus, including weight and height should be noted.

At the initial examination, blood pressure should be measured in both arms and preferably in the supine, sitting and standing positions to evaluate for postural hypotension.

Arterial pressure should be measured at least once in the lower extremity in patients in whom hypertension is discovered before age of 30 years.

Heart rate also should be recorded.

The neck should be palpated for an enlarged thyroid gland, and patients should be assessed for signs of hypo- and hyperthyroidism.

Examination of Blood Vessels

- Visible arterial pulsations—Suprasternal and neck region
- Include funduscopic examination
- Auscultation for bruits over the carotid, renal and femoral arteries
- Palpation of peripheral pulses.

Apical Impulse

Left ventricular hypertrophy—Enlarged, sustained and laterally displaced apical impulse.

Examination of the Heart

A loud A_2 due to closure of the aortic valve an S_4 gallop attributed to atrial contraction against a noncompliant left ventricle.

Palpable Kidneys

In polycystic kidney disease.

Complications

Cerebrovascular

Ischemic stroke and intracerebral hemorrhage, hypertensive encephalopathy and dementia.

Hypertensive heart disease—Left ventricular hypertrophy (LVH), coronary artery disease, cardiac arrhythmias (specially atrial fibrillation) and congestive heart failure (CHF).

Hypertensive emergencies—Acute pulmonary edema, hypertensive encephalopathy, intracranial hemorrhage, aortic dissection, eclampsia and acute myocardial infarction.

Investigations

Tests described in Table 38.2 are used for investigation of systemic hypertension.

Table 38.2: Investigations

Test
Microalbuminuria, serum creatinine, blood urea and uric acid
Serum sodium, potassium, calcium and thyroid stimulating hormone (TSH)
Fasting blood glucose and lipid profile
Hematocrit, ECG, chest radiograph and echocardiogram (when indicated)

Treatment (Table 38.3)

Table 38.3: Nonpharmacological methods

Nonpharmacological methods—Lifestyle modifications	
Weight reduction	Attain and maintain BMI <25 kg/m^2
Dietary salt reduction	<6 gm NaCl/day
	Diet rich in fruits, vegetables, and low-fat dairy products with reduced content of saturated and total fat
Moderation of alcohol consumption	For those who drink alcohol, consume 2 drinks/day in men and 1 drink/day in women
Physical activity	Regular aerobic activity, e.g. brisk walking for 30 minutes/day

Pharmacological Treatment

Pharmacological therapy used to treat systemic hypertension is described in Table 38.4.

Table 38.4: Pharmacological treatment

BP classification	SBP* mmHg	DBP** mmHg	Lifestyle modification	Initial drug therapy	
				Without compelling indication	With compelling indication
Normal	<120	<80	Encourage	No antihypertensive drug indicated	Drug(s) for compelling indications
Prehypertension	120–139	80–89	Yes		
Stage 1 hypertension	140–159	90–99	Yes	Thiazide-type diuretics for most. It may consider ACEI, ARB, BB, CCB, or combination	Drug(s) for the compelling indications. Other antihypertensive drugs (diuretics, ACEI, ARB, BB and CCB) as needed
Stage 2 hypertension	>/=160	>/= 100	Yes	Two-drug combination for most (usually thiazide-type diuretic and ACEI or ARB or BB or CCB)	

*SBP—Systolic BP
**DBP—Diastolic BP

Medication Selection Based on Joint National Committee 8 (JNC8) (Table 38.5)

Table 38.5: Medication based on JNC8

Patient characteristics	Initial treatment
Nonblack	Thiazide CCB ACEI ARB
Black	Thiazide CCB
CKD	ACEI ARB

Chapter 39

Ischemic Heart Disease

Definition

Ischemic heart disease (IHD) is a condition in which there is an inadequate supply of blood and oxygen to a portion of the myocardium.

Microvascular angina—Abnormal constriction or failure of normal dilation of the coronary resistance vessels can cause cause angina.

Major risk factors for atherosclerosis are high levels of LDL, low HDL, cigaret smoking, hypertension and diabetes mellitus.

Prinzmetal's angina—Pathologic spasm of coronaries precipitate myocardial ischemia.

Stable Angina Pectoris

- This episodic clinical syndrome is due to transient myocardial ischemia.
- Males constitute ~70% of all patients with angina pectoris.
- The typical patient with angina is a man >50 years or a woman >60 years of age.
- Complaints—Episodes of chest discomfort, usually described as heaviness.
- Patient typically places a hand over the sternum to describe central, substernal discomfort (Levine's sign).
- Angina is usually crescendo-decrescendo in nature, typically lasts 2–5 minutes, and can radiate to either shoulder or to both arms (specially the ulnar surfaces of the forearm and hand).
- It also can arise in or radiate to the back, interscapular region, root of the neck, jaw, teeth and epigastrium.
- Although episodes of angina typically are caused by exertion (exercise, hurrying, or sexual activity) or emotion (stress, anger, fright, or frustration) and are relieved by rest, they also may occur at rest (unstable angina pectoris) and while the patient is recumbent (angina decubitus) (Table 39.1).

- Exertional angina typically is relieved in 1–5 minutes by slowing or ceasing activities and even more rapidly by rest and sublingual nitroglycerin.

Table 39.1: NYHA classification

Class	New York Heart Association Functional Classification
I	Patients have cardiac disease but without resulting limitations of physical activity. Ordinary physical activity does not cause undue fatigue, palpitation, dyspnea, or anginal pain
II	Patients have cardiac disease resulting in slight limitation of physical activity. They are comfortable at rest. Ordinary physical activity results in fatigue, palpitation, dyspnea, or anginal pain
III	Patients have cardiac disease resulting in marked limitation of physical activity. They are comfortable at rest. Less than ordinary physical activity causes fatigue, palpitation, dyspnea, or anginal pain
IV	Patients have cardiac disease resulting in inability to carry on any physical activity without discomfort. Symptoms of cardiac insufficiency or of the anginal syndrome may be present even at rest. If any physical activity is undertaken, discomfort is increased

Anginal "Equivalents"

- These are symptoms of myocardial ischemia other than angina
- Include dyspnea, nausea, fatigue and faintness
- More common in the elderly and in diabetic patients.

Physical Examination

- The physical examination is often normal in patients with stable angina.
- Search for evidence of atherosclerotic disease at other sites, such as an abdominal aortic aneurysm, carotid arterial bruits and diminished arterial pulses in the lower extremities.
- Search for evidence of risk factors for atherosclerosis such as xanthelasmas and xanthomas.
- Examination of the fundi may reveal an increased light reflex and arteriovenous nicking as evidence of hypertension.
- Signs of anemia, thyroid disease and nicotine stains on the fingertips from cigaret smoking.
- Palpation may reveal cardiac enlargement and abnormal contraction of the cardiac impulse (left ventricular dyskinesia).
- Auscultation can uncover arterial bruits, S_3 and S_4.
- If acute ischemia or previous infarction has impaired papillary muscle function, there is an apical systolic murmur due to mitral regurgitation.

Laboratory Examination

Lipid profile, fasting plasma glucose, hemoglobin A1c, creatinine, hematocrit and thyroid function.

Chest X-ray

- Cardiac enlargement
- Ventricular aneurysm
- Signs of heart failure.

Elevated level of high-sensitivity C-reactive protein (CRP) (specifically, between 0 and 3 mg/dL) is an independent risk factor for ischemic heart disease (IHD).

Electrocardiogram

- Evidence of an old myocardial infarction
- ST-segment and 'T' wave changes
- Left ventricular hypertrophy
- Disturbances of cardiac rhythm.

Stress Testing

- Most widely used test for diagnosis of IHD.
- Estimation of risk and prognosis.
- Involves recording the 12-lead ECG before, during and after exercise, usually on a treadmill.
- The test consists of a standardized incremental increase in external workload while symptoms, the ECG and arm blood pressure are monitored.
- The test is discontinued upon evidence of chest discomfort, severe shortness of breath and ST-segment depression > 2 mm.
- This test is used to discover any limitation in exercise performance, detect typical ECG signs of myocardial ischemia, and establish their relationship to chest discomfort.
- The ischemic ST-segment response generally is defined as flat or downsloping depression of the ST-segment >1 mm below baseline and lasting longer than 0.08 seconds.
- Stress myocardial radionuclide perfusion imaging (after the intravenous administration of thallium-201 or 99m technetium sestamibi) or positron emission tomography (PET) imaging during exercise.

Echocardiography

- Assess left ventricular function in patients with chronic stable angina and with a history of a prior myocardial infarction, pathologic 'Q' waves, or clinical evidence of heart failure.

- Two-dimensional echocardiography can assess both global and regional wall motion abnormalities of the left ventricle.
- Stress (exercise or dobutamine) echocardiography may cause the emergence of regions of akinesis or dyskinesis.
- Cardiac MRI can be used to provide more complete ventricular evaluation.

Coronary Arteriography
- It is used to detect or exclude serious coronary obstruction.
- Coronary arteriography is indicated in patients with chronic stable angina pectoris who are severely symptomatic despite medical therapy and are being considered for revascularization, i.e. percutaneous coronary intervention (PCI) or coronary artery bypass grafting (CABG).

Treatment
Treatment of stable angina pectoris:
1. Explanation and reassurance.
2. Identification and treatment of aggravating conditions and risk factors.
   - Left ventricular hypertrophy, aortic valve disease and hypertrophic cardiomyopathy should be excluded or treated.
   - Obesity, hypertension, dyslipidemia and diabetes should be treated aggressively.
   - Avoid cigaret smoking.
   - A diet low in saturated and trans unsaturated fatty acids and a reduced caloric intake to achieve optimal body weight are a cornerstone in the management of chronic IHD.
   - HMG-CoA reductase inhibitors (statins) are required and can lower LDL cholesterol, raise HDL cholesterol and lower triglycerides.
   - Fibrates or niacin can be used to raise HDL cholesterol and lower triglycerides.
3. Adaptation of activity
   - Many tasks that ordinarily evoke angina may be accomplished without symptoms simply by reducing the speed at which they are performed.
   - On occasion, it may be necessary to recommend a change in employment or residence to avoid physical stress.
   - A regular program of isotonic exercise that is within the limits of the individual patient's threshold are recommended for the development of angina pectoris.

4. Drug therapy
   - Nitrates—Nitroglycerin (sublingual, spray, oral, IV and transdermal), isosorbide dinitrate, isosorbide mononitrate and pentaerythritol tetranitrate.
   - β-blockers—Metoprolol, bisoprolol, atenolol and nebivolol.
   - Calcium channel blockers—Dihydropyridines (amlodipine and nifedipine) and nondihydropyridines (diltiazem and verapamil).
   - Antiplatelet drugs
     - Aspirin has been shown to reduce coronary events in patients with chronic stable angina, and patients who have or have survived unstable angina and myocardial infarction.
     - It is preferable to use an enteric-coated formulation in the range of 81–162 mg/day.
     - Clopidogrel combined with aspirin reduces death and coronary ischemic events in patients with an acute coronary syndrome and also reduces the risk of thrombus formation in patients undergoing implantation of a stent in a coronary artery.
     - Alternative antiplatelet agents that block the P2Y12 platelet receptor-prasugrel.
   - ACE inhibitors
     The benefits of ACE inhibitors are most evident in IHD patients at increased risk, specially if diabetes mellitus or LV dysfunction is present.
   - Ranolazine may be useful for patients with chronic angina despite standard medical therapy.
   - Agents that open ATP-sensitive potassium channels—Nicorandil.
5. Coronary revascularization— It is of two types, PCI or CABG.

Revascularization should be considered in the presence of unstable phases of the disease, intractable symptoms, severe ischemia or high-risk coronary anatomy, diabetes and impaired LV function.

Asymptomatic (Silent) Ischemia

Obstructive CAD, acute myocardial infarction and transient myocardial ischemia are frequently asymptomatic. Patients with asymptomatic ischemia after a myocardial infarction are at greater risk for a second coronary event. The widespread use of exercise ECG during routine examinations has also identified some of these previously unrecognized patients with asymptomatic CAD.

Chapter 40

ST-segment Elevation Myocardial Infarction (STEMI)

Introduction
- When patients with prolonged ischemic discomfort at rest are first seen, the working clinical diagnosis is that they are suffering from an acute coronary syndrome.
- The 12-lead electrocardiogram (ECG) permits distinction of those patients presenting with ST-segment elevation from those presenting without ST-segment elevation.
- Serum cardiac biomarkers distinguish unstable angina (UA) from non-ST-segment MI (NSTEMI) and to assess the magnitude of an ST-segment elevation MI (STEMI).

Pathophysiology
- Slowly developing, high-grade coronary artery stenoses do not typically precipitate STEMI because of the development of a rich collateral network over time.
- Instead, STEMI occurs when a coronary artery thrombus develops rapidly at a site of vascular injury.

Clinical Presentation
- A precipitating factor may be present before STEMI, such as vigorous physical exercise, emotional stress, or a medical or surgical illness.
- It is seen more in the morning within a few hours of awakening.
- Pain is the most common presenting complaint.
- The pain is deep and visceral.
- Heavy, squeezing and crushing pain.
- It is usually more severe and lasts longer than anginal pain.
- Typically, the pain involves the central portion of the chest and/or the epigastrium.
- It radiates to the arms.

- Less common sites of radiation include the abdomen, back, lower jaw and neck.
- It is often accompanied by weakness, sweating, nausea, vomiting, anxiety and a sense of impending doom.
- Painless STEMI is greater in patients with diabetes mellitus and it increases with age.
- In the elderly, STEMI may present as sudden-onset of breathlessness, which may progress to pulmonary edema.

Physical Findings

- Patients are anxious and restless.
- Pallor associated with perspiration.
- The combination of substernal chest pain persisting for >30 minutes and diaphoresis strongly suggests STEMI.
- About one-fourth of patients with anterior infarction have manifestations of sympathetic nervous system hyperactivity (tachycardia and/or hypertension).
- Upto one-half of the patients with inferior infarction show evidence of parasympathetic hyperactivity (bradycardia and/or hypotension).
- The precordium is usually quiet.
- Physical signs of ventricular dysfunction include fourth and third heart sounds, decreased intensity of the first heart sound, and paradoxical splitting of the second heart sound.
- A transient apical systolic murmur due to dysfunction of the mitral valve apparatus may be present.
- A pericardial friction rub is heard in many patients with transmural STEMI.
- Temperature elevations upto 38°C during the first week after STEMI.
- In most patients with transmural infarction, systolic pressure declines by approximately 10–15 mmHg from the preinfarction state.

Laboratory Findings

Electrocardiogram

- In the initial stage, total occlusion of an epicardial coronary artery produces ST- elevation.
- Then T invertion occurs.
- Q waves evolve later denoting transmural MI (Fig. 40.1).

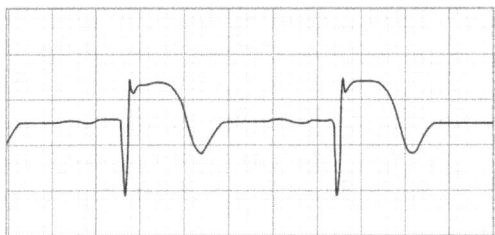

Fig. 40.1: ECG in acute myocardial infarction

Serum Cardiac Biomarkers

Troponin

1. Cardiac-specific troponin T (cTnT) and cardiac-specific troponin I (cTnI).
2. Of particular value in distinguishing UA from NSTEMI.
3. Levels of cTnI and cTnT may remain elevated for 7–10 days after STEMI.

Creatine Kinase

- Creatine kinase (CK) rises within 4–8 hours.
- Generally returns to normal by 48–72 hours.
- Its lack of specificity for STEMI, as CK may be elevated with skeletal muscle disease or trauma, including intramuscular injection.
- The MB isoenzyme of CK is considerably more specific.
- Cardiac surgery, myocarditis and electrical cardioversion often result in elevated CK-MB.
- A ratio of CK-MB mass: CK activity of 2.5 suggests a myocardial source.
  1. The nonspecific reaction to myocardial injury is polymorphonuclear leukocytosis.
  2. The white blood cell count often reaches levels of 12,000–15,000/liter.
  3. The erythrocyte sedimentation rate peaks during the first week.

Chest X-ray

- Hilar haziness is seen if pulmonary edema present
- Cardiomegaly is present in long-standing hypertension.

Cardiac Imaging

- Abnormalities of wall motion are viewed on two-dimensional echocardiography.
- Echocardiographic estimation of left ventricular (LV) function (ejection fraction) is useful prognostically.
- Echocardiography may also identify the presence of right ventricular (RV) infarction, ventricular aneurysm, pericardial effusion and LV thrombus.

- Doppler echocardiography is useful in the detection of a ventricular septal defect and mitral regurgitation, which are two serious complications of STEMI.
- Myocardial perfusion imaging with (201 thallium) or [99m technetium]-sestamibi, reveal a defect ("cold spot") in most patients during the first few hours after development of a transmural infarct.

Initial Management

Aspirin

- It is effective across the entire spectrum of acute coronary syndromes.
- Rapid inhibition of cyclo-oxygenase-1 in platelets followed by reduction of thromboxane A_2 (TXA_2) levels.
- It is achieved by buccal absorption of a chewed 160–325 mg tablet.
- It should be followed by daily oral administration of aspirin in a dose of 75–162 mg.

Oxygen

When hypoxemia is present, O_2 should be administered by nasal prongs or face mask (2–4 liter/minute) for the first 6–12 hours after infarction.

Control of discomfort

Sublingual nitroglycerin— Upto 3 doses of 0.4 mg should be administered at about 5 minute intervals.

Morphine

- It is a very effective analgesic for the pain associated with STEMI.
- Morphine is routinely administered by repetitive (every 5 minute) intravenous injection of small doses (2–4 mg).

Intravenous β-blockers

- These are also useful in controlling the pain of STEMI.
- Metoprolol, 5 mg every 5 minute for a total of 3 doses.
- Fifteen minutes after the last intravenous dose, an oral regimen is initiated of 50 mg every 6 hour for 48 hours, followed by 100 mg every 12 hour.

Management Strategies

- When ST-segment elevation of at least 2 mm in two contiguous precordial leads and 1 mm in two adjacent limb leads is present, a patient should be considered a candidate for reperfusion therapy.
- Reperfusion in patients with STEMI can be accomplished by the pharmacologic (fibrinolysis) or catheter-based (primary PCI) approaches.

Limitation of Infarct Size

- Timely restoration of flow in the epicardial infarct-related artery combined with improved perfusion of the downstream zone of infarcted myocardium results in a limitation of infarct size.
- Glucocorticoids and nonsteroidal anti-inflammatory agents, with the exception of aspirin, should be avoided in patients with STEMI. They can impair infarct healing and increase the risk of myocardial rupture, and their use may result in a larger infarct scar.

Percutaneous coronary intervention (PCI) (Fig. 40.2)

Usually angioplasty and/or stenting without preceding fibrinolysis, referred to as primary PCI, is effective in restoring perfusion in STEMI when carried out on an emergency basis in the first few hours of MI.

Fibrinolysis

- Fibrinolytic therapy should ideally be initiated within 30 minutes of presentation (i.e. door-to-needle time—30 minutes).
- The principal goal of fibrinolysis is prompt restoration of full coronary arterial patency. The fibrinolytic agents tissue plasminogen activator (t-PA), streptokinase, tenecteplase (TNK) and reteplase (rPA) act by promoting the conversion of plasminogen to plasmin, which subsequently lyses fibrinthrombi.
- TNK and rPA are referred to as bolus fibrinolytics since their administration does not require a prolonged intravenous infusion.
- Fibrinolytic therapy appears to reduce infarct size, limit LV dysfunction, and reduce the incidence of serious complications such as septal rupture and cardiogenic shock.
- The therapy remains of benefit for 3–6 hours after the onset of infarction, and some benefit appears to be possible upto 12 hours.
- Facilitated PCI—Fibrinolytic agent is given as part of a preparatory regimen before planned immediate PCI.
- Clear contraindications to the use of fibrinolytic agents include a history of cerebrovascular hemorrhage at any time, a nonhemorrhagic stroke

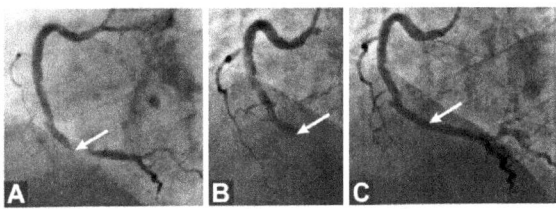

Fig. 40.2: PCI

within the past year, marked hypertension (>180/110 mmHg), aortic dissection and active internal bleeding (excluding menses).
- Relative contraindications to fibrinolytic therapy—Use of anticoagulants, a recent surgical procedure, prolonged (>10 minutes) cardiopulmonary resuscitation, known bleeding diathesis, pregnancy and active peptic ulcer disease.
- Because of the risk of an allergic reaction, patients should not receive streptokinase if that agent had been received within the preceding 5 days to 2 years.

Thrombolysis in Myocardial Infarction (TIMI) Grading

When assessed angiographically, flow in the culprit coronary artery is described by TIMI grading system:
- Grade 0 indicates complete occlusion.
- Grade 1 indicates some penetration of the contrast material.
- Grade 2 indicates perfusion of the entire infarct vessel, but with delayed flow.
- Grade 3 indicates full perfusion of the infarct vessel with normal flow.

Patients who have a confirmed STEMI but who are considered to be at low-risk—No persistent chest discomfort, CHF, hypotension, or cardiac arrhythmias may be transferred out of the coronary care unit within 24 hours.

Activity

- Patients with STEMI should be kept at bed rest for the first 12 hours.
- By the second or third day ambulation should be started with increasing duration and frequency.

Sedation

Diazepam (5 mg) or lorazepam (0.5–2 mg), given 3–4 times daily, is usually effective.

Pharmacotherapy

Antithrombotic agents

- The addition of the P2Y12 inhibitor clopidogrel to background treatment with aspirin to STEMI patients reduces the risk of clinical events.
- New P2Y12 ADP receptor antagonists, such as prasugrel and ticagrelor, are more effective than clopidogrel.
- The standard anticoagulant agent used in clinical practice is unfractionated heparin (UFH).

- The recommended dose of UFH is an initial bolus of maximum 4000 U followed by an initial infusion of maximum 1000 U/hour.
- Alternatives to UFH are the low-molecular-weight heparin (LMWH) preparations—Enoxaparin, fondaparinux and bivalirudin.
- Anticoagulant therapy is indicated in AWMI, severe LV dysfunction, heart failure, a history of embolism, echo evidence of mural thrombus, or atrial fibrillation. Heparin followed by at least 3 months of warfarin therapy.

β-Adrenoceptor Blockers

Acute intravenous β-blockade improves the myocardial O_2 supply-demand relationship, decreases pain, reduces infarct size and decreases the incidence of serious ventricular arrhythmias.

ACE Inhibitors

- Reduce the mortality rate after STEMI
- Reduction in ventricular remodeling after infarction.

Angiotensin Receptor Blockers (ARBs)

- It should be administered to STEMI patients who are intolerant of ACE inhibitors.
- Who have either clinical or radiological signs of heart failure.

Complications and their Management

Ventricular dysfunction

- After STEMI, the left ventricle undergoes changes in shape, size and thickness in both the infarcted and noninfarcted segments—Ventricular remodeling.
- Progressive dilation may be ameliorated by therapy with ACE inhibitors and other vasodilators (e.g. nitrates).
- In patients with an ejection fraction <40%, ACE inhibitors or ARBs should be prescribed.
- The most common clinical signs are pulmonary rales and S_3 and S_4 gallop sounds. Pulmonary congestion is also frequently seen on the chest roentgenogram.
- Elevated LV filling pressure and elevated pulmonary artery pressure are the characteristic hemodynamic findings.

Killip Classification

- Class I—No signs of pulmonary or venous congestion.

- Class II—Moderate heart failure as evidenced by rales at the lung bases, S_3 gallop.
- Class III—Severe heart failure and pulmonary edema.
- Class IV—Shock.

Cardiogenic Shock

Patients who develop cardiogenic shock have severe multivessel coronary artery disease.

Right Ventricular Infarction

- Approximately one-third of patients with inferior infarction demonstrate RVMI.
- Clinically significant RV infarction causes signs of severe RV failure— Jugular venous distension, Kussmaul's sign and hepatomegaly with or without hypotension.
- ST-segment elevations of right-sided precordial ECG leads, particularly lead V4R.
- Therapy consists of volume expansion to maintain adequate RV preload.

Arrhythmias

Most deaths from arrhythmia occur during the first few hours after infarction.

Ventricular Arrhythmias

- Ventricular premature beats
- Ventricular tachycardia and fibrillation
- Accelerated idioventricular rhythm.

Supraventricular Arrhythmias

- Sinus tachycardia is the most common supraventricular arrhythmia.
- Other common arrhythmias in this group are atrial flutter and atrial fibrillation.
- Digoxin is usually the treatment of choice for supraventricular arrhythmias if heart failure is present.

Sinus Bradycardia

- Atropine is given intravenously in doses of 0.5 mg initially.
- Upto a total of 2.0 mg, may be given.
- Persistent bradycardia (<40 bpm) despite atropine may be treated with electrical pacing.

Atrioventricular and Intraventricular Conduction Disturbances

For example, complete atrioventricular (AV) block.

Other Complications
- Recurrent chest discomfort—Post MI angina.
- Dressler's syndrome—Pericarditis secondary to MI.
- Thromboembolism.
- Left ventricular aneurysm.
- In stable patients, submaximal exercise stress testing may be carried out before hospital discharge.
- Alternatively a maximal (symptom-limited) exercise stress test may be carried out 4–6 weeks after infarction.
- Evaluation of LV function by echocardiography is usually warranted.

Cardiac catheterization with coronary angiography is indicated in
- When angina is induced at low workloads
- Depressed ejection fraction
- Those with demonstrable ischemia
- Exercise provokes symptomatic ventricular arrhythmias.

The usual duration of hospitalization for an uncomplicated STEMI is about 5 days. Most patients will be able to return to work within 2–4 weeks.

Secondary Prevention
- Long-term treatment with an antiplatelet agent usually aspirin 75–150 mg/day.
- An alternative antiplatelet agent for patients intolerant of aspirin is clopidogrel (75 mg orally daily).
- ACE inhibitors or ARBs should be used indefinitely by patients with clinically evident heart failure, a moderate decrease in global ejection fraction, or a large regional wall motion abnormality to prevent late ventricular remodeling and recurrent ischemic events.
- The chronic routine use of oral β-adrenoceptor blockers is indicated for at least 2 years after STEMI.
- Add warfarin for patients at increased risk of embolism.
- Atorvastatin 80 mg daily should be started immediately post MI period.

Chapter 41

Unstable Angina and Non-ST-segment Elevation Myocardial Infarction

Definition

Stable angina pectoris is characterized by chest discomfort associated with physical exertion or stress and is relieved within 5–10 minutes by rest and/or sublingual nitroglycerin.

Unstable angina is defined as angina pectoris with at least one of three features:

1. It occurs at rest, usually lasting >10 minutes
2. It is severe and of new onset
3. It occurs with a crescendo pattern (more severe, prolonged, or frequent).

NSTEMI

In a patient with the clinical features of UA develops evidence of myocardial necrosis, as reflected in elevated cardiac biomarkers.

Clinical Presentation

- History and physical examination.
- Chest pain, typically located in the substernal region or sometimes in the epigastrium.
- Radiates to the neck, left shoulder, and/or the left arm.
- Anginal "equivalents" such as dyspnea and epigastric discomfort may also occur.
- The physical examination may be unremarkable.
- The physical findings can include diaphoresis; pale, cool skin; sinus tachycardia; a third and/or fourth heart sound; basilar rales; and sometimes hypotension.

Electrocardiogram

- ST-segment depression

- Transient ST-segment elevation
- 'T' wave inversion.

Cardiac Biomarkers

- Elevated levels of CK-MB and troponins distinguish patients with NSTEMI from UA.
- There is a direct relationship between the degree of troponin elevation and mortality.

Four major diagnostic tools are used in the diagnosis of UA/NSTEMI:
- Clinical history
- The ECG
- Cardiac markers
- Stress testing.

Medical Treatment

- Bed rest.
- Continuous ECG monitoring for ST-segment deviation and cardiac arrhythmias.

Anti-ischemic treatment

It is given to provide relief and prevention of recurrence of chest pain, initial treatment should include bed rest, nitrates and β-blockers.

Nitrates

- Nitrates should first be given sublingually or by buccal spray
- If pain persists, intravenous nitroglycerin is recommended
- Topical or oral nitrates can be used once the pain has resolved.

β-adrenergic blockers—Oral β-blockade targeted to a heart rate of 50–60 beats/minute is recommended as first-line treatment—Metoprolol 50 mg 6th hourly.

Morphine

It is given when symptoms are not relieved by sublingual nitroglycerin.

Nondihydropyridine calcium channel blockers

Heart rate—Slowing calcium channel blockers, e.g. verapamil or diltiazem, are recommended for patients who have persistent symptoms after treatment with nitrates and β-blockers.

Additional medical therapy includes angiotensin-converting enzyme (ACE) inhibitors and HMG-CoA reductase inhibitors (statins) for long-term secondary prevention.

Early administration of intensive statin therapy (e.g. atorvastatin 80 mg) is also included for treatment.

Antithrombotic Therapy

Aspirin

- Initial treatment should begin with the platelet cyclooxygenase inhibitor aspirin.
- The typical initial dose is 325 mg/day.
- Lower doses (75–162 mg/day) recommended for long-term therapy.

Clopidogrel

- The thienopyridine, clopidogrel blocks the platelet P2Y12 or the ADP receptor.
- Pretreatment with clopidogrel includes a 300 or 600 mg loading dose, followed by 75 mg/day.
- Dual antiplatelet(clopidogrel and aspirin) should be continued for 1 year.

Anticoagulant Therapy

- This has to be added to aspirin and clopidogrel.
- Unfractionated heparin (UFH) is the mainstay of therapy.
- The low-molecular-weight heparin (LMWH) or enoxaparin, has been shown to be superior to UFH in reducing recurrent cardiac events. Indirect factor Xa inhibitor, fondaparinux or bivalirudin, or a direct thrombin inhibitor may be used alternatively.

Invasive Strategy

- Multiple clinical trials have demonstrated the benefit of an early invasive strategy in high-risk patients.
- In this strategy, following treatment with anti-ischemic and antithrombotic agents, coronary arteriography is carried out within 48 hours of admission, followed by coronary revascularization (PCI or coronary artery bypass grafting).

Conservative Strategy

- This strategy is applied in low-risk patients.
- It consists of anti-ischemic and antithrombotic therapy.
- In this strategy coronary arteriography is carried out only if rest pain or ST-segment changes recur.

Long-term Management
- Risk-factor modification—Smoking cessation, achieving optimal weight, daily exercise following an appropriate diet, blood pressure control, tight control of hyperglycemia (for diabetic patients) and lipid management.
- β-blockers, statins (at a high dose, e.g. atorvastatin 80 mg/day) and ACE inhibitors or angiotensin receptor blockers are recommended for long-term plaque stabilization.
- Antiplatelet therapy, now recommended to be the combination of aspirin and clopidogrel for 1 year, with aspirin continued thereafter.

Prinzmetal's Variant Angina
- In 1959, Prinzmetal described the syndrome.
- Severe ischemic pain that occurs at rest but not usually with exertion and is associated with transient ST-segment elevation.
- Due to focal spasm of an epicardial coronary artery leading to severe myocardial ischemia.
- Generally younger patients have fewer coronary risk factors (with the exception of cigaret smoking).
- Detection of transient ST-segment elevation with rest pain.
- Many patients exhibit multiple episodes of asymptomatic ST-segment elevation (silent ischemia).
- Small elevations of troponin may occur in patients with prolonged attacks of variant angina.
- Coronary angiography demonstrates transient coronary spasm as the diagnostic hallmark.
- Focal spasm is most common in the right coronary artery.
- Nitrates and calcium channel blockers are the main agents used to treat acute episodes.
- Aspirin may actually increase the severity of ischemic episodes, as a result of the exquisite sensitivity of coronary tone to modest changes in the synthesis of prostacyclin.
- The response to β-blockers is variable.
- Nonfatal MI occurs in upto 20% of patients by 5 years.

Chapter 42

Arrhythmias

Tachyarrhythmias

Tachyarrhythmias are defined as heart rhythms with a rate in excess of 100 beats/minute further be classified into:
- Supraventricular tachycardia (origin above the bifurcation of bundle of His).
- Ventricular tachycardia.

Arrhythmias can be also be classified morphologically into:
- Narrow complex tachycardia (duration of QRS < 120 msec, i.e. 3 small squares in ECG).
- Wide complex tachycardia (duration of QRS > 120 msec).

Analysis of ECG for Arrhythmia

Look for:
- Frequency, morphology and regularity of 'P' waves
- Sinus 'P' wave/ectopic P/flutter wave/fibrillation wave
- Relationship between atrial and ventricular activity
- QRS morphology during sinus rhythm/tachyarrhythmia
- Response to carotid sinus massage/vagal maneuvers.
- Atrial tachycardia—200 ± 50 beats/minute
- Atrial flutter—300 ± 50 beats/minute
- Atrial fibrillation—400 ± 50 beats/minute
- Ventricular tachycardia—200 ± 50 beats/minute.

Paroxysmal Supraventricular Tachycardia (Fig. 42.1)

- Reentry is responsible for the majority of SVT.
- Anatomical site has been localized to the sinus node, atrium, AV node or a macroentry circuit involving AV node and AV bypass tract.

- The mechanism of paroxysmal supraventricular tachycardia (PSVT) can be traced on the basis of R-P interval, the time interval between the peak of an 'R' wave and the subsequent 'P' wave during tachycardia.

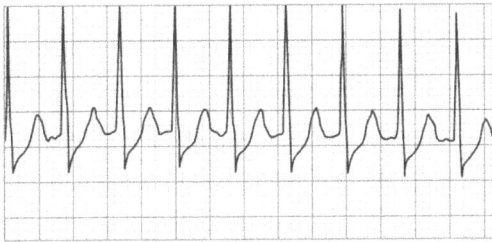

Fig. 42.1: ECG in PSVT

Short R-P tachycardia

They have an R-P interval that is less than 50% of the R-R interval. These include:
  a. Typical AV nodal reentrant tachycardia (AVNRT):
     - Conduction proceeds antegradely down the slow pathway and retrograde conduction up the fast pathway resulting in atrial and ventricular excitation concurrently. 'P' waves are hidden within the QRS complexes.
  b. Orthodromic AV reentrant tachycardia:
     - It is an accessory pathway mediated reentrant rhythm
     - 'P' waves are seen shortly after QRS complexes.
  c. Sinus tachycardia or ectopic atrial tachycardia with first degree AV block.
  d. Junctional tachycardia:

It is a narrow complex tachycardia arising from the AV junction. The impulse is conducted to the atrium and ventricle simultaneously and the 'P' wave is not easily discernible. It is seen in acute MI, digitalis toxicity.

Long R-P tachycardia

They have an R-P interval that is greater than 50% of the R-R interval.

WPW syndrome (Fig. 42.2)

Pre-excitation is as a result of anterograde activation of the ventricle via an accessory pathway as well as the AV node, resulting in a short P-R interval with a delta wave slurring the upstroke of the QRS complex.

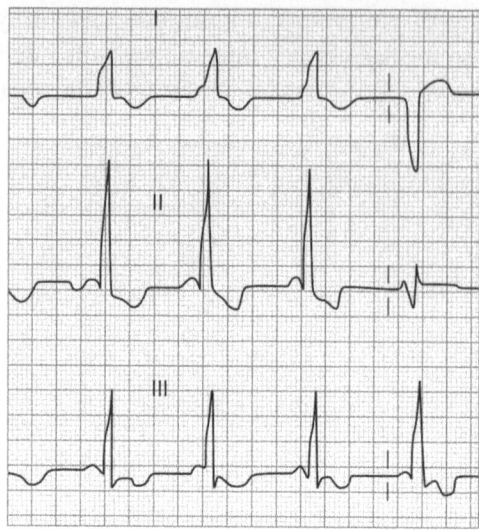

Fig. 42.2: ECG in WPW syndrome

The presence of accessory pathway predisposes the individuals for SVT.

Multifocal atrial tachycardia

Multifocal atrial tachycardia is revealed by 3 or more varying 'P' wave morphologies with irregular QRS complexes. This tachycardia is commonly seen in COPD patients specially when on theophylline.

Paroxysmal atrial tachycardia with complete heart block

This is a manifestation specific for digoxin toxicity.

Atrial Flutter (Fig. 42.3)

- Result of single reentrant circuit around conduction barriers (scar due to prior cardiac surgery) within the atria.

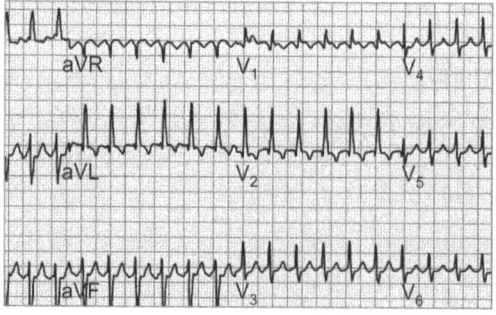

Fig. 42.3: ECG in atrial flutter

- Flutter waves are negative in inferior leads (II, III and aVF) and positive in V_1 with 'sawtooth' appearance.
- Atrial rate is usually 300 beats/minute.

Atrial Fibrillation (Fig. 42.4)

It is the most common and sustained tachyarrhythmia seen in many patients.

Common causes

- 10% of elderly > 75 years
- Lone AF— < 65 years (normotensive with normal heart)
- Valvular heart disease
- Hypertensive heart disease
- Coronary artery disease
- Myocarditis and cardiomyopathy
- Cardiac surgery
- Hypothyroidism
- Hyperthyroidism
- Pheochromocytoma
- Pericarditis.

Atrial rate is 400–600 beats/minute with irregularly irregular rapid ventricular rate (> 100 beats/minute).

ECG

- Absent 'P' waves
- Varying R-R interval.

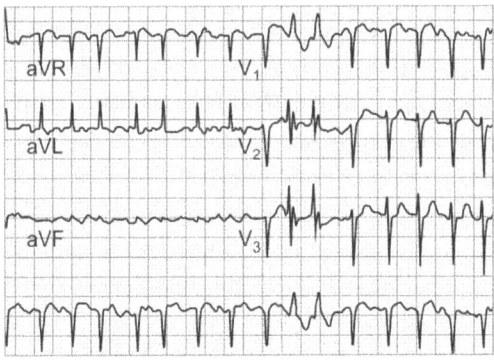

Fig. 42.4: ECG in AF

Symptoms of AF (due to rapid ventricular rate)

1. Acute pulmonary edema
2. Syncope

3. Angina
4. Palpitations
5. Thromboembolic (cerebral, peripheral, renal and coronary).

Management of Narrow Complex Tachycardia

Vagal maneuvers such as Valsalva maneuver, carotid sinus massage, eyeball compression and tickling the fauces.

If it fails, administer IV bolus of drugs that block AV nodal conduction. either of the followings:

- Adenosine (drug of choice) 6 mg IV and repeat if necessary every 2 minutes using 12 mg.
- Verapamil 5 mg IV(over 3 minutes) and repeat after 15 minutes or metoprolol 5 mg IV every 5 minutes.
- Diltiazem.
- Esmolol.
- Digoxin maximum IV dose 0.5 mg over 3 minutes.
- Amiodarone IV infusion 300 mg over 1 hour.
- Overdrive pacing.

In the presence of adverse signs like

- Hypotension—BP < 90 mmHg
- Acute severe chest pain
- Heart failure
- Altered conscious level
- Heart rate > 200 beats/minute.
  1. Give sedation and synchronized cardioversion.
  2. Amiodarone 150 mg IV over 10 minutes and then 300 mg over 1 hour.

Chronic Therapy of SVT (Use Either One of the Drugs)

- Diltiazem
- Verapamil
- Metoprolol
- Atenolol
- Digoxin.

Radiofrequency Ablation after Electrophysiological Study

It offers definitive cure for different type of SVTs
1. AVNRT/AVRT
2. Accessory pathway mediated tachycardias
3. Focal atrial tachycardia
4. Atrial flutter.

Atrial Fibrillation: Management

Acute AF (< 72 hours)

- Treat the associated acute illness
- Control ventricular rate with β-blocker, and/or calcium channel blockers — verapamil or diltiazem.
- Drug—Cardioversion can be tried with either amiodarone or flecainide.
  Amiodarone: 5 mg/kg over 1 hour, then 100 mg over 2 hours with central line, then:
    - PO 200 mg tid in the first week
    - 200 mg bid second week
    - 100–200 mg od for maintenance.

DC—Cardioversion is indicated electively following the first attack of AF with an identifiable cause and as an emergency if the patient is compromised (200 Joules biphasic shock is typically used for cardioversion).

Anticoagulation with warfarin is essential for 3 weeks before and 4 weeks after cardioversion to prevent thromboembolic episodes.

Paroxysmal AF

Use either
1. Sotalol
2. Amiodarone.

Chronic AF

1. Digoxin is the ideal drug to control the ventricular rate.
2. Amiodarone is the most effective antiarrhythmic agent for the maintenance of sinus rhythm.
3. Anticoagulation is not required if AF is of recent onset with structurally normal heart on echocardiography, but aspirin may be given.
4. In all other cases of AF, anticoagulation with warfarin should be given.

It is further categorized as AF with high and moderate risk factors.

AF with High Risk Factors

- Age greater than 75 years
- Previous stroke or TIA
- Systemic embolus
- Valvular heart disease
- Poor LV systolic function.

AF with Moderate Risk Factors

- Age between 65–75 years
- Diabetes mellitus
- Hypertension

- CAD with normal LV function.

Use warfarin to keep the INR 2–3 in patients with one high risk factor or more than 2 moderate risk factors. Warfarin is not indicated for patients without risk factors and in them, use aspirin 325 mg od.

Atrial Flutter

- Management is similar to AF including anticoagulation
- If drugs fail, consider 'cavotricuspid isthmus' ablation.

Atrial Extrasystoles

- This is characterized by the presence of a bizarre 'P' wave
- The width of the QRS complex is normal
- The compensatory pause is relative.

AV Node

AV nodal extrasystole

This is similar in appearance to atrial extrasystole on the ECG.

Paroxysmal AV nodal tachycardia

- This may be defined as a succession of three or more AV nodal extrasystoles.
- It has similar characteristics as that of atrial tachycardia.

Ventricular Arrythmias

Ventricular extrasystole

- It is also known as ventricular ectopics and ventricular premature contractions (VPC).
- Appearance of a premature and bizarre (widened and slurred or notched) QRS complex, with associated secondary ST-T changes (ST-segment is depressed and 'T' wave is inverted).
- The ventricular extrasystole is followed by an absolute compensatory pause.
- Ventricular ectopics may be benign, due to excessive ingestion of coffee, tea, alcohol, cold water, smoking, or emotional stress.
- Ventricular ectopics with a predominant negative QRS deflection in the right precordial leads (V_1, V_2) indicate that ectopics originate from RV, and are usually benign.
- Ectopics with predominant negative QRS deflection, in the left precordial leads (V_4, V_5, V_6) indicate that ectopics originate from LV and are usually pathological.
- Stoppage of precipitating factors and use of β-blockers form the mainstay of treatment.

Types of Ventricular Extrasystole

Ventricular bigeminy (Fig. 42.5)

- Extrasystoles which occur after every other sinus beat, are the most common cause of bigeminal rhythm.
- A frequent manifestation of digitalis intoxication.

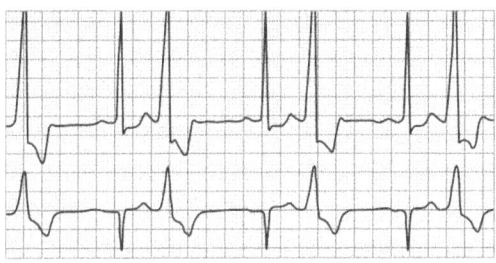

Fig. 42.5: ECG in ventricular bigeminy

Multifocal ventricular extrasystoles

Extrasystoles that arise from different foci and consequently give rise to different QRS complexes.

Ventricular trigeminy

A sinus beat followed by two extrasystoles.

Ventricular extrasystoles are always significant when associated with myocardial disease.

Frequent ventricular extrasystoles, specially those occurring in pairs, often heralded as ventricular tachycardia or ventricular fibrillation.

Broad complex tachycardia—Ventricular tachycardia (VT)

Characteristics suggestive of VT
- AV dissociation
- Fusion beats
- Capture beats
- Left bundle branch block (LBBB) morphology with right axis deviation
- QRS morphology suggestive of VT.
- **Sustained Monomorphic VT**—Three or more successive ventricular premature complexes are termed ventricular tachycardia. It is called sustained when it lasts longer than 30 seconds at a rate of 100–250 beats/minute with only 1 type QRS morphology throughout the arrhythmia.

Polymorphic VT

- It is characterized by changing QRS morphology from beat to beat and is frequently due to coronary artery disease.

Ventricular Flutter (Fig. 42.6)

- Heart rate—150–300 beats/minute.
- ECG shows very rapid and regular ectopic ventricular discharge. The QRS and T deflections are very wide and bizarre, resulting in a sine-like waveform.

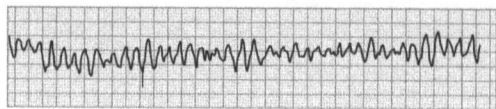

Fig. 42.6: ECG in ventricular flutter

Torsades de pointes

- Ventricular flutter may present with multiform QRS complexes.
- The QRS complexes tend to be bizarre and multiform and have sharply pointed apices.
- This is frequently associated with syncopal attacks resulting in marked prolongation of the QTc interval and there may be 'giant 'T' wave inversion'.
- It may be seen in severe coronary artery disease, hypokalemia, hypomagnesemia and quinidine therapy.

Ventricular Fibrillation (VF) (Fig. 42.7)

This is characterized in the ECG by the presence of completely irregular, chaotic and deformed deflections of varying height, width and shape.

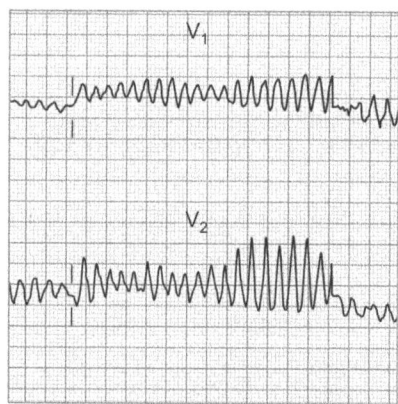

Fig. 42.7: ECG in ventricular fibrillation

Management of Broad Complex Tachycardia

Hemodynamically stable VT

1. Correct hypokalemia and hypomagnesemia.
2. Amiodarone 150 mg IV over 20 minutes and then 300 mg over 1 hour or

lignocaine 50 mg IV over 2 minutes and repeated every 5 minutes to a maximum of 200 mg.
3. If the above drugs fail or the patient hemodynamically unstable: DC cardioversion is given (200 Joules followed by 200 Joules followed by 360 Joules).

Resistant VT/ VF
- Amiodarone 300 mg IV followed by an infusion 1 mg/minute for 6 hours and then 0.5 mg/minute for another 6 hours or lignocaine 100 mg IV—Repeat once more, followed by infusion 2–4 mg/minute.
- Procainamide, bretylium and sotalol may also be used.

Torsades de Pointes (Tdp) is Associated With Long QT Syndrome
- Immediate DC cardioversion
- Magnesium sulfate IV bolus 1–2 gm.

Prevention of Recurrent VT
- Radiofrequency catheter ablation of VT for hemodynamically stable forms of VT without structural heart disease.
- Surgical isolation of arrhythmogenic area.
- Implantation of tiny automatic defibrillators.

Indications for Implantable Cardioverter Defibrillators (ICDs)
- Spontaneous VT with structural heart disease
- Irreversible causes for VT/VF
- Recurrent VT/VF
- Failure of antiarrhythmic agents to control VT
- Patients with high risk for sudden cardiac death(SCD).

Bradyarrhythmias

Sick Sinus Syndrome (Tachy-Brady Syndrome)
- This is due to sinus node dysfunction.
- ECG shows sinus bradycardia, sometimes associated with AV nodal block.
- It may be associated with tachycardias such as PSVT and atrial fibrillation.
- Sick sinus syndrome is more common in elderly adults, due to scar-like degeneration of the cardiac conduction system.

Heart Block

First degree heart block
- It is characterized by a constantly prolonged PR interval (> 0.20 second) (Fig. 42.8).

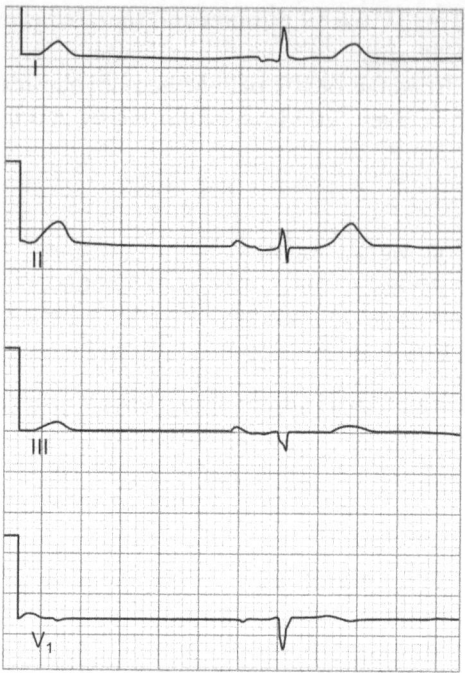

Fig. 42.8: ECG in 1st degree heart block

Second degree heart block

Second degree heart block are of 2 types:

a. Mobitz type I (Wenckebach's phenomenon)—The P-R interval is prolonged till a QRS complex is missed (Fig. 42.9).

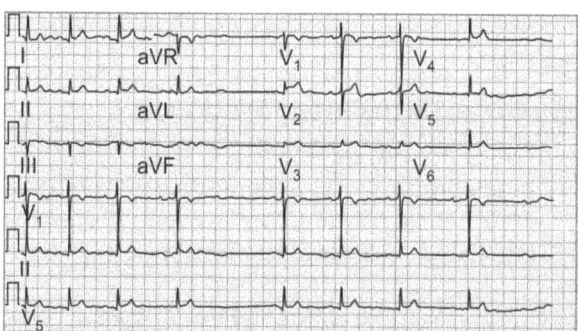

Fig. 42.9: ECG in Wenckebach's phenomenon

b. Mobitz type II (Fig. 42.10)
   1. The P-R interval is constant
   2. Some 'P' waves are not followed by a QRS complex
   3. The degree of block can be 2:1 or 3:1.

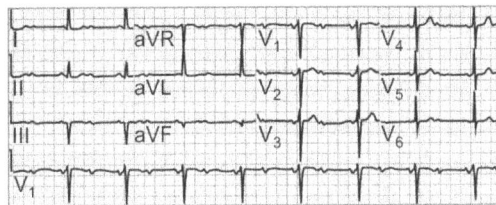

Fig. 42.10: ECG in Mobitz type II heart block

Complete or third degree heart block (Fig. 42.11)
- It is characterized by 'P' waves and the QRS complexes occurring completely independent of each other.
- ECG—Constant P-P interval and R-R interval. Varying P-R interval.

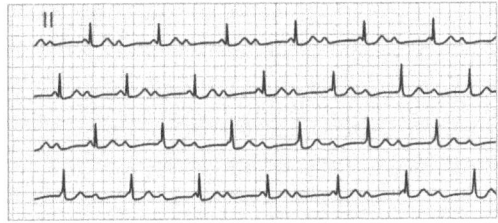

Fig. 42.11: ECG in complete heart block

Administration of 1–2 mg of atropine IV does not increase heart rate in sick sinus syndrome and complete heart block, whereas heart rate increases in sinus bradycardia and first or second degree heart block.

Indications for Permanent Pacemakers
- Symptomatic sinus bradycardia or AV block
- Advanced AV block with asystole > 3 seconds
- Neuromuscular disorders
- Postoperative AV block (recovery remote)
- Extreme degree of sinus bradycardia due to drug therapy
- Complete heart block
- Type II second degree block.

Exercise (Stress) ECG

By performing an ECG during progressively increasing exercise (on a treadmill), it is possible to detect stress-induced arrhythmia or evidence of ischemia.

Predicted Heart Rate

It is 220—Age of the patient, following MI, it is used in assessing the risk.

Holter Monitoring or Ambulatory ECG

Holter monitoring is done for detecting transient episodes of arrhythmia or ischemia.

Stress Echocardiography

A stress echocardiography can be done following administration of adenosine, dobutamine or dipyridamole to detect evidence of ischemia.

Chapter 43

Conduction Disorders of the Heart

Conduction pathway

Signals arising in the SA node stimulate the atria to contract and travel to the AV node. After a delay, the stimulus is conducted through the bundle of His to the Purkinje fibers and the endocardium at the apex of the heart, then finally to the ventricular epicardium.

Right Bundle Branch Block (RBBB) (Fig. 43.1)

Complete RBBB

- Wide 'S' wave in LI, V_5 and V_6
- In V_1, tall, wide-notched 'R' wave
- QRS duration > 0.12 second in V_1 and V_2.

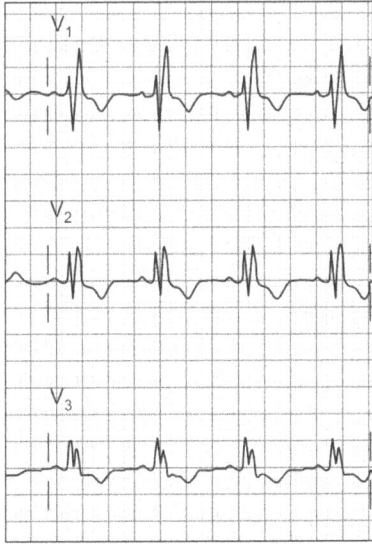

Fig. 43.1: ECG in RBBB

Incomplete RBBB

- Diminution of 'S' wave in V_2 (earliest sign of RBBB)
- QRS duration < 0.12 second
- RSR pattern in V_1 and V_2.

Significance

- RBBB may be physiological.
- It may also occur with CAD, ASD, cardiomyopathy and massive pulmonary embolism.
- RBBB, RAD and RVH go together.

Left Bundle Branch Block (LBBB) (Fig. 43.2)

Complete LBBB

a. Prolonged QRS duration > 0. 12 second.
b. There should be a QS or rS complex in lead V_1.
c. There should be an RSR' wave in lead V_6.
d. Secondary S-T, T changes opposite in direction to terminal QRS deflection.
e. 'T' wave discordance—'T' wave is deflected opposite the terminal deflection of the QRS complex.
f. A concordant 'T' wave may suggest ischemia or myocardial infarction.

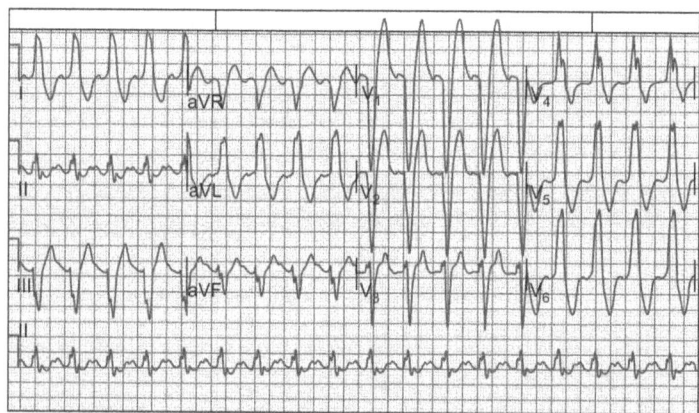

Fig. 43.2: ECG in LBBB

Significance

LBBB indicates organic heart disease. It is commonly seen in IHD or hypertensive heart disease.

Hemiblocks (Fascicular Blocks)

Left Anterior Hemiblock (LAHB) (Fig. 43.3)

Causes

- Coronary artery disease
- Cardiomyopathy
- Longstanding systemic hypertension
- Longstanding CCF.

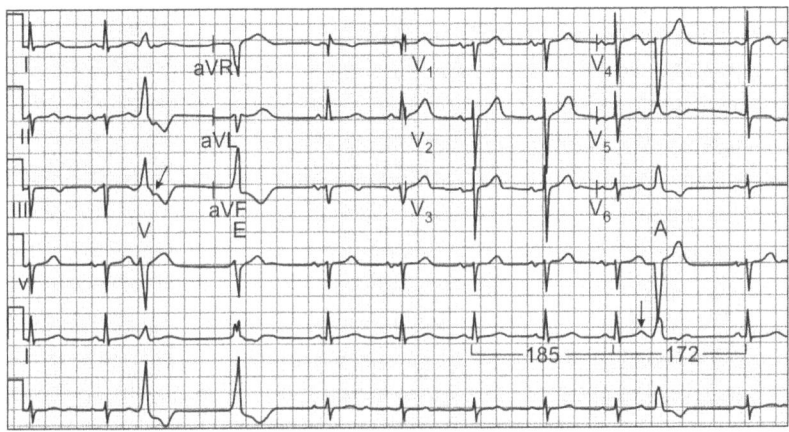

Fig. 43.3: ECG in LAHB

ECG features

1. Left axis deviation.
2. rS complex in lead II.
3. Lead I and aVL—Prominent initial 'Q' wave followed by a ensuing tall 'R' wave.
4. Lead aVR—Late and slurred terminal 'R' wave.
5. Lead V_5 and V_6—No initial 'Q' waves, attenuation of 'R' waves and prominence of 'S' waves.
6. 'T' waves are in opposite direction to the main QRS deflection.

Left anterior hemiblock (LAHB) when occurs in association with RBBB, it usually indicates a poor prognosis and may lead to complete AV block. When it occurs with LBBB, prognosis is worse.

Left Posterior Hemiblock (LPHB) (Fig. 43.4)

Occurrence of LPHB is very rare.

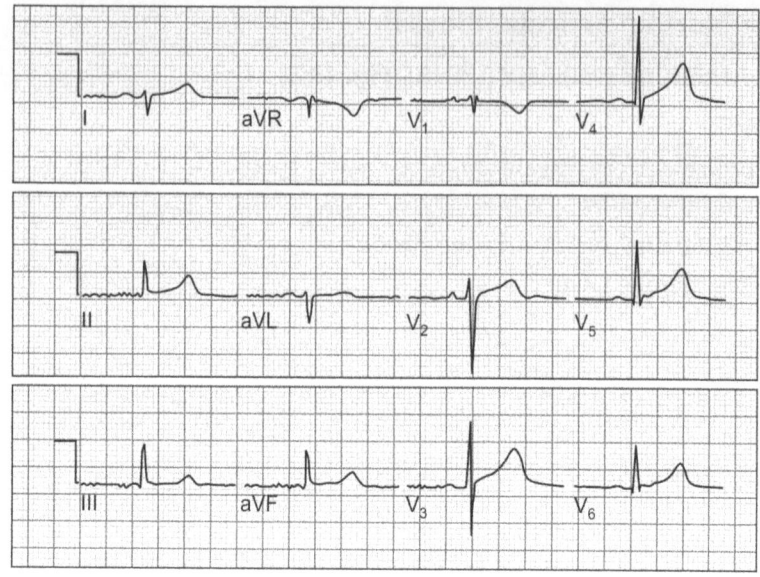

Fig. 43.4: ECG is LPHB

ECG features

- Right axis deviation
- Prominent small initial 'Q' waves in lead II, III and aVF
- A small initial 'R' wave in lead I
- The distal limb of the tall 'R' wave in lead III is notched
- Inverted 'T' waves in leads II, III and aVF
- Upright 'T' waves in lead I.

LPHB with sinus tachycardia may denote pulmonary embolism.

Bifascicular Block

It is the combination of RBBB and left bundle hemiblock.

Trifascicular Block

It is the combination of bifascicular block and first degree heart block.

Chapter 44

Pericardial Diseases

Pericarditis

Acute < 6 weeks
- Fibrinous
- Effusive.

Subacute 6 weeks–6 months
- Effusive
- Constrictive.

Chronic > 6 months
- Constrictive
- Effusive
- Adhesive.

Etiologic Classification

Infectious pericarditis
- Viral
- Pyogenic
- Tuberculous
- Mycotic
- Syphilitic.

Noninfectious pericarditis
- Acute MI
- Uremia
- Neoplasia (primaries and secondaries)
- Myxedema

- Chylopericardium
- Trauma
- Postirradiation
- Infectious mononucleosis
- Familial pericarditis
- Sarcoidosis
- Idiopathic
- Familial mediterranean fever
- Aortic aneurysm with leak into pericardium.

Pericarditis Related to Hypersensitivity or Autoimmunity

1. Rheumatic fever
2. Collagen vascular disorders
   - Systemic lupus erythematosus (SLE)
   - Rheumatoid arthritis
   - Scleroderma
3. Drug-induced
   - Procainamide
   - Hydralazine
   - Isoniazid (INH)
   - Minoxidil
4. Postcardiac injury
   - After MI (Dressler's syndrome)
   - Postpericardiotomy.

There are four principal diagnostic features

Chest pain
- Severe, retrosternal and left precordial and referred to the neck, arms, or left shoulder.
- Often the pain is pleuritic, resembles that of myocardial ischemia.
- Pericardial pain is relieved by sitting up and leaning forward.
- Pain is intensified by lying supine.

A pericardial friction rub
- It may have upto 3 components per cardiac cycle.
- It is high-pitched.
- It is described as rasping, scratching, or grating.
- It can be elicited when the diaphragm of the stethoscope is applied firmly to the chest wall at the left-lower sternal border.

- It is heard most frequently at end expiration with the patient upright and leaning forward.
- The rub is often inconstant, and the loud to and fro leathery sound.
- A pericardial rub is heard throughout the respiratory cycle, whereas a pleural rub disappears when respiration is suspended.

ECG (Fig. 44.1)

There is widespread elevation of the ST-segments, often with upward concavity.

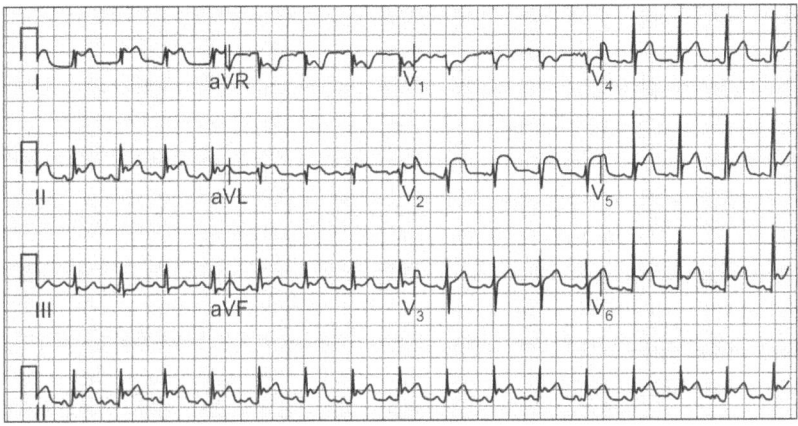

Fig. 44.1: ECG in pericarditis

Pericardial effusion

- Pericardial effusion is specially important clinically when it develops within a relatively short time as it may lead to cardiac tamponade.
- Heart sounds may be fainter with pericardial effusion.
- The friction rub may disappear.
- The apex impulse remains palpable medial to the left border of cardiac dullness.
- The base of the left lung may be compressed by pericardial fluid, producing Ewart's sign, a patch of dullness and increased fremitus beneath the angle of the left scapula.
- The chest roentgenogram may show a "water bottle" configuration of the cardiac silhouette.

Management

1. Aspirin or indomethacin are useful. When the response is not satisfactory, steroids can be used.
2. Anticoagulants are contraindicated (hemopericardium or tamponade may occur).

3. Steroids are best avoided in pericarditis following MI because of myocardial aneurysm formation and rupture.
4. In chronic pericarditis, pericardiectomy should be considered.
5. Treatment of the cause.

Cardiac Tamponade

The accumulation of fluid in the pericardium sufficient to cause serious obstruction to the inflow of blood to the ventricles results in cardiac tamponade.

Causes

- Neoplastic disease
- Idiopathic pericarditis
- Uremia
- Tuberculosis
- Cardiac surgery
- Trauma
- Hemopericardium.

Clinical Features

- The symptoms depend upon the rapidity of accumulation of fluid.
- As small as 200 mL can produce the critical state when fluid develops rapidly or more than 2 liters in slowly developing effusions.
- Patient presents with severe dyspnea, chest tightness and dizziness.
- Paradoxical pulse—It consists of a greater than normal (10 mmHg) inspiratory decline in systolic arterial pressure. When severe, it may be detected by palpating disappearance of the arterial pulse during inspiration.
- Beck's triad—
  1. Hypotension
  2. Raised JVP— A prominent 'x' descent but an absent 'y' descent
  3. Muffled or absent heart sounds.
- ECG.
- Low voltage complexes with or without electrical alternans.
- Echocardiogram.
- Diastolic collapse of RV-free wall and RA is the characteristic feature of cardiac tamponade.

Management

- Pericardiocentesis must be carried out at once and is life-saving.
- Surgical drainage through a limited thoracotomy in recurrent tamponade.

Chronic Constrictive Pericarditis

Causes

- Tuberculous
- Trauma
- Cardiac surgery
- Mediastinal irradiation
- Histoplasmosis
- Neoplastic disease (breast cancer, lung cancer and lymphoma)
- Rheumatoid arthritis and SLE
- Chronic renal failure with uremia.

Pathology

Obliteration of the pericardial cavity with the formation of granulation tissue. The latter gradually contracts and forms a firm scar, which may be calcified, encasing the heart and interfering with filling of the ventricles.

In constrictive pericarditis, the ventricular pressure pulses in both ventricles exhibit characteristic "square root" signs during diastole.

Clinical and Laboratory Findings

- Weakness, fatigue, weight gain, increased abdominal girth, abdominal discomfort, a protuberant abdomen and edema are common.
- The patient appears chronically ill.
- In advanced cases there are anasarca, skeletal muscle wasting and cachexia.
- Exertional dyspnea and orthopnea may occur, although it is usually not severe.
- JVP may remain elevated even after intensive diuretic treatment.
- Absence of inspiratory fall in jugular venous pressure (Kussmaul's sign).
- The pulse pressure is normal or reduced.
- In about one-third of cases, a paradoxical pulse can be detected.
- Congestive hepatomegaly may impair hepatic function and cause jaundice.
- Ascites is common and is usually more prominent than dependent edema.
- The apical pulse is reduced and may retract in systole (Broadbent's sign).
- The heart sounds may be distant.
- An early third heart sound is often conspicuous.
- A systolic murmur of tricuspid regurgitation may be present.

- The ECG—Low voltage of the QRS complexes and diffuse inversion of the 'T' waves.
- Atrial fibrillation is present in about one-third of patients.
- The chest roentgenogram shows a normal or slightly enlarged heart.
- Pericardial calcification is most common in tuberculous pericarditis.
- Echocardiogram typically shows pericardial thickening.
- MRI and CT scanning are more accurate.

Differential Diagnosis

- Tricuspid stenosis
- Restrictive cardiomyopathy
- Right ventricular endomyocardial fibrosis (RVEMF).

Treatment of Chronic Constrictive Pericarditis

- Initial treatment—Dietary sodium restriction and diuretics are useful.
- Pericardial resection is the only definitive treatment of constrictive pericarditis.

Chapter 45

Myocarditis

Definition

Myocarditis is the inflammation of myocardium.

Causes

Infective

Bacterial

- *Staphylococcus aureus* endocarditis
- Diphtheria
- Lyme disease (tick-borne spirochete)
- *Salmonella*
- Tuberculosis
- β-hemolytic streptococci
- Meningococci
- Leptospirosis.

Viral

- Coxsackie B virus
- HIV
- Influenza
- Poliomyelitis
- Hepatitis C virus and adenovirus
- Cytomegalovirus
- Epstein-Barr virus.

Fungal

- Candida
- Cryptococci

- Blastomyces
- Aspergillus.

Rickettsia

- *Rickettsia typhi* (typhus)
- *Rickettsia tsutsugamushi* (scrub typhus).

Chlamydia

- *C. psittaci*.

Protozoal

- Trypanosomiasis
- Toxoplasmosis.

Hypersensitivity

Acute rheumatic fever.

Physical agents

- Radiation
- Heat stroke.

Chemicals

- Cobalt
- Antimony
- Arsenic.

Drugs

- Phenothiazines
- Tricyclic antidepressants
- Emetine
- Penicillin
- Methyldopa.

Myocarditis may progress to dilated cardiomyopathy.

Clinical Features

- Fatigue
- Angina
- Dyspnea
- Disproportionate tachycardia
- Heart failure.

On Examination

- Muffled S_1

- S_3
- MR murmur
- Pericardial friction rub.

ECG
- Disproportionate tachycardia
- Transient ST-T changes
- Atrial or ventricular ectopics.

Diagnosis
By clinical features and identification of causative organisms.

Management
- No strenuous activity.
- Management of arrhythmias.
- Specific antimicrobial therapy or antitoxin.
- Avoid nonsteroidal anti-inflammatory drugs (NSAIDs) as they may worsen myocardial damage.
- Effectiveness of steroid therapy is controversial.

Chapter 46

Cardiomyopathy

Cardiomyopathies are primary disorders of heart muscle.

Types of Cardiomyopathy

There are 3 types of cardiomyopathy. These are—Dilated cardiomyopathy, restrictive cardiomyopathy and hypertrophic obstructive cardiomyopathy.

Dilated Cardiomyopathy

There is impaired ventricular contraction leading to progressive left-sided and later right-sided failure. There may be functional MR or TR. Systolic failure is more marked than the diastolic dysfunction.

Table 46.1: Causes of dilated cardiomyopathy

Inflammatory myocarditis
Infective 1. Viral (coxsackie, adenovirus, HIV and hepatitis C) 2. Parasitic (*T. cruzi*—Chagas disease and toxoplasmosis) 3. Bacterial (diphtheria) 4. Spirochetal (*Borellia burgdorferi*—Lyme disease) 5. Rickettsial—*Q fever* 6. Fungal (with systemic infection)
Noninfective 1. Granulomatous inflammatory disease 2. Sarcoidosis 3. Giant cell myocarditis 4. Hypersensitivity myocarditis 5. Polymyositis and dermatomyositis 6. Collagen vascular disease 7. Peripartum cardiomyopathy

Contd...

Contd...

Toxic 1. Alcohol 2. Amphetamines and cocaine 3. Chemotherapeutic agents: Anthracyclines and trastuzumab 4. Hydroxychloroquine and chloroquine
Metabolic
Nutritional deficiencies: Thiamine, selenium and carnitine
Endocrinopathy 1. Thyroid disease 2. Pheochromocytoma 3. Diabetes
Hemochromatosis
Dystrophin-related dystrophy (Duchenne's and Becker's)
Mitochondrial myopathies (e.g. Kearns-Sayre syndrome)
Overlap with restrictive cardiomyopathy
Hemochromatosis
Amylodosis

Clinical Features
Exertional dyspnea and fatigue.

ECG
Nonspecific; ST-T wave changes are seen.

Chest X-ray
Flask-shaped heart (Fig. 46.1).

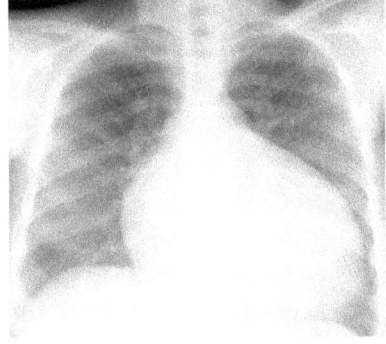

Fig. 46.1: X-ray chest in dilated cardiomyopathy

Echocardiography

Global hypokinesia and dilated heart (LV dilatation).

Cardiac Catheterization

- LV dilatation and dysfunction
- Increased left and right-sided filling pressures
- Decreased cardiac output.

Management

1. Antifailure measures
2. Consider heart transplant
3. Anticoagulants
4. Avoid NSAIDs, alcohol and calcium channel blockers.

Restrictive (Obliterative) Cardiomyopathy

There is impairment of ventricular filling because they are stiff. This leads to high atrial pressure, hypertrophy and dilatation of atria and atrial fibrillation.

Causes

- Endomyocardial fibrosis
- Constrictive pericarditis
- Eosinophilic heart muscle disease
- Amyloidosis.

Chest X-ray

Mild cardiomegaly.

ECG

- Low voltage
- Conduction defects.

Doppler Echocardiography

- Abnormal diastolic function
- Symmetrical thickened LV walls
- A normal systolic function.

CT and MRI

Detect thickened pericardium in constrictive pericarditis.

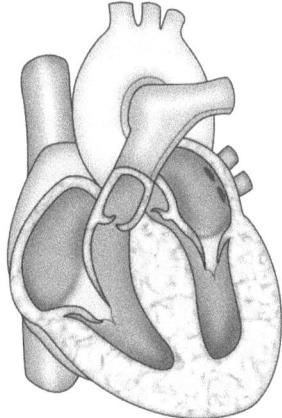

Fig. 46.2: Hypertrophic obstructive cardiomyopathy

Endomyocardial Biopsy

Interstitial infiltration or fibrosis.

Hypertrophic Obstructive Cardiomyopathy (HCM) (Fig. 46.2)

- It can be familial (autosomal dominant) or sporadic.
- In familial cases, abnormality of β-myosin heavy chain gene on chromosome 14 is found.
- Asymmetric hypertrophy of septum (ASH).
- Systolic anterior motion of anterior leaflet of mitralvalve (SAM).
- Stiff, noncompliant ventricle impedes diastolic filling.
- Dynamic LV outflow tract obstruction and MR.

Symptoms

- Dyspnea
- Angina
- Syncope
- Palpitation
- Sudden death.

Signs

- Jerky pulse
- Double or triple apical impulse
- S_3
- S_4
- Late systolic murmur
- AF common.

ECG
- LVH
- LBBB
- Deep broad 'Q' waves
- Arrhythmias [Superior ventricular tachycardia (SVT), AF and VT].

Chest X-ray
Mild to moderate cardiac enlargement.

Echocardiography
- Asymmetric hypertrophy of septum (ASH)
- Systolic anterior motion of anterior leaflet of mitral valve (SAM).

Cardiac Catheterization
- Small, banana-like or spade-shaped LV cavity
- Thickened papillary muscle and trabeculae
- Cavity obliteration in systole
- Dynamic LV outflow obstruction.

Management
- β-blocker for angina.
- Amiodarone for arrhythmia.
- Septal myectomy or myotomy.
- In chronic AF and anticoagulation.
- Avoid diuretics, digitalis, β-agonists, nitrates and vasodilators like nifedipine.
- IE prophylaxis when associated with MR.
- Alcohol ablation treatment.
- Insertion of an implantable cardioverter defibrillator in high risk patients.
- Verapamil and diltiazem.

Sudden death is common in those who have—
  i. Ventricular tachycardia (nonsustained)
  ii. Family history of sudden death.

Chapter 47

Diseases of the Aorta

Aortic Aneurysm

- An aneurysm is defined as a pathologic dilation of a segment of a blood vessel.
- A true aneurysm involves all three layers of the vessel wall.
- A pseudoaneurysm, in which the intimal and medial layers are disrupted and the dilated segment of the aorta is lined by adventitia only.

Classification Aneurysms

According to their Gross Appearance

- Fusiform aneurysm
- Saccular aneurysm.

According to Location (Fig. 47.1)

- Abdominal
- Thoracic
- Thoracoabdominal.

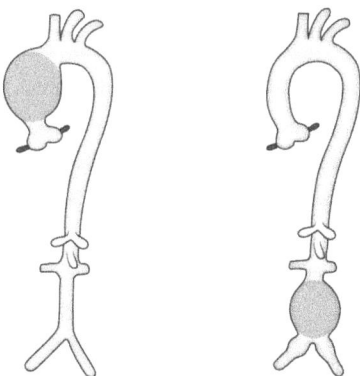

Fig. 47.1: Classification of aneurysms based on location

Etiology (Table 47.1)

Table 47.1: Etiology of aortic aneurysm

Aortic aneurysm • Degenerative/atherosclerosis • Aging • Male gender • Family history • Cystic medial necrosis • Marfan syndrome • Ehlers-Danlos syndrome • Familial • Bicuspid aortic valve • Chronic aortic dissection • Infective—Syphilis, tuberculosis and mycotic • Trauma
Aortic dissection • Atherosclerosis • Cystic medial necrosis • Hypertension • Vasculitis • Pregnancy • Trauma
Aortic occlusion • Atherosclerosis • Thromboembolism

Aortitis
1. Vasculitis
   • Takayasu's arteritis
   • Giant cell arteritis
2. Rheumatic
   • HLA-B27—Associated spondyloarthropathies
   • Behçet's syndrome
   • Cogan's syndrome
3. Idiopathic aortitis
4. Infective—Syphilis, tuberculosis and mycotic

- Approximately 90% of syphilitic aneurysms are located in the ascending aorta or aortic arch.
- Tuberculous aneurysms typically affect the thoracic aorta.
- Marfan syndrome affect the thoracic aorta.
- Takayasu's arteritis and giant cell arteritis cause aneurysms of aortic arch and descending thoracic aorta.

Thoracic Aortic Aneurysms

- Most thoracic aortic aneurysms are asymptomatic.

- Compression or erosion of adjacent tissue by aneurysms cause symptoms such as chest pain, shortness of breath, cough, hoarseness, and dysphagia.
- Oliver's sign or the tracheal tug sign is an abnormal downward movement of the trachea during systole that indicate an aneurysm of the aortic arch.

Chest X-ray
- Widening of the mediastinal shadow
- Compression of the trachea or left mainstem bronchus.

Transesophageal Echocardiography

It can be used to assess the proximal ascending aorta and descending thoracic aorta.

Contrast-enhanced CT, magnetic resonance imaging (MRI) and invasive aortography are used for assessment of aneurysms of the thoracic aorta.

Treatment

Operative repair with placement of a prosthetic graft.

Abdominal Aortic Aneurysms

- It occurs more frequently in males.
- Incidence increases with age.
- Abdominal aortic aneurysms >4.0 cm are related to atherosclerotic disease.
- Most of these aneurysms are below the level of the renal arteries.
- An abdominal aortic aneurysm commonly produces no symptoms.
- A palpable, pulsatile, expansile and nontender mass.
- As abdominal aortic aneurysms expand, they may become painful.
- Aneurysmal pain is usually a harbinger of rupture.
- Acute pain and hypotension occur with rupture of aneurysm, which requires an emergency operation.
- Abdominal radiography may demonstrate the calcified outline of the aneurysm.
- An abdominal ultrasound can delineate the dimensions of aneurysm.
- CT with contrast and MRI are accurate noninvasive tests.

Treatment

Operative repair of the aneurysm with insertion of a prosthetic graft or an aortic stent graft.

Aortic Dissection

- It is caused by a circumferential or transverse tear of the intima.
- Thoracic aortic dissections are of 2 types namely, DeBakey and Stanford.
- The peak incidence of aortic dissection is in the sixth and seventh decades.
- Men are more affected.
- Acute aortic dissection presents with the sudden onset of tearing pain.
- The pain may be localized to the front or back of the chest, often the interscapular region.
- Other symptoms include syncope and dyspnea.
- Physical findings may include hypertension or hypotension, loss of pulses and aortic regurgitation.
- Neurologic findings are carotid artery obstruction (hemiplegia) or spinal cord ischemia (paraplegia).
- Bowel ischemia, hematuria and myocardial ischemia have been observed.
- For acute dissection, intravenous metoprolol or esmolol is used to achieve a heart rate of 60 beats/minute.
- Sodium nitroprusside infusion is used to lower systolic blood pressure to ≤120 mmHg.
- Urgent surgical correction is the preferred treatment.

Aortitis

Caused by—
  a. Large vessel vasculitides such as Takayasu's arteritis and giant cell arterities.
  b. Rheumatic and HLA-B_{27} associated spondyloarthropathies.
  c. Behcet's syndrome.
  d. Antineutrophil cytoplasmic antibodies (ANCA) associated vasculitides.
  e. Cogan's syndrome.
  f. Infections like syphilis, tuberculosis and Salmonella.
  g. May be associated with retroperitoneal fibrosis.

Aortitis may result in aneurysmal dilation and aortic regurgitation, occulusion of the aorta and its branch vessels, or acute aortic syndromes.

Takayasu's Arteritis

This inflammatory disease often affects the ascending aorta and aortic arch, causing obstruction of the aorta and its major arteries. Takayasu's arteritis is also termed pulseless disease because of the frequent occlusion of the large arteries originating from the aorta. It also may involve the descending thoracic and abdominal aorta and occlude large branches such as the renal arteries. Aortic aneurysms also may occur. The pathology is a panarteritis characterized by mononuclear cells and occasionally giant cells, with marked intimal hyperplasia, medial and adventitial thickening and, in the chronic form, fibrotic occlusion. The disease is most prevalent in young females of Asian descent but does occur in women of other geographic and ethnic origins and also in young men. During the acute stage, fever, malaise, weight loss and other systemic symptoms may be evident. Elevations of the erythrocyte sedimentation rate and C-reactive protein are common. The chronic stages of the disease, which is intermittently active, present with symptoms related to large artery occlusion, such as upper extremity claudication, cerebral ischemia and syncope. The process is progressive and there is no definitive therapy. Glucocorticoids and immunosuppressive agents have been reported to be effective in some patients during the acute phase. Surgical bypass or endovascular intervention of a critically stenotic artery may be necessary.

Giant Cell Arteritis

This vasculitis occurs in older individuals and affects women more often than men. Primarily large- and medium-size arteries are affected. The pathology is that of focal granulomatous lesions involving the entire arterial wall; it may be associated with polymyalgia rheumatica. Obstruction of medium-size arteries (e.g. temporal and ophthalmic arteries) and major branches of the aorta and the development of aortitis and aortic regurgitation are important complications of the disease. High-dose glucocorticoid therapy may be effective when given early.

Rheumatic Aortitis

Rheumatoid arthritis, ankylosing spondylitis, psoriatic arthritis, reactive arthritis (formerly known as Reiter's syndrome), relapsing polychondritis and inflammatory bowel disorders may all be associated with aortitis involving the ascending aorta. The inflammatory lesions usually involve the ascending aorta and may extend to the sinuses of Valsalva, the mitral valve leaflets and adjacent myocardium. The clinical manifestations are aneurysm, aortic regurgitation and involvement of the cardiac conduction system.

Idiopathic Aortitis

Idiopathic abdominal aortitis is characterized by adventitial and periaortic inflammation with thickening of the aortic wall. It is associated with abdominal aortic aneurysms and idiopathic retroperitoneal fibrosis. Affected individuals may present with vague constitutional symptoms, fever and abdominal pain. Retroperitoneal fibrosis can cause ureteral obstruction and hydronephrosis. Glucocorticoids and immunosuppressive agents may reduce the inflammation.

Infective Aortitis

Infective aortitis may result from direct invasion of the aortic wall by bacterial pathogens such as *Staphylococcus, Streptococcus* and *Salmonella* or by fungi. These bacteria cause aortitis by infecting the aorta at sites of atherosclerotic plaque. Bacterial proteases lead to degradation of collagen, and the ensuing destruction of the aortic wall leads to the formation of a saccular aneurysm referred to as a mycotic aneurysm. Mycotic aneurysms have a predilection for the suprarenal abdominal aorta. The pathologic characteristics of the aortic wall include acute and chronic inflammation, abscesses, hemorrhage and necrosis. Mycotic aneurysms typically affect the elderly and occur in men three times more frequently than in women. Patients may present with fever, sepsis and chest, back, or abdominal pain; there may have been a preceding diarrheal illness. Blood cultures are positive in the majority of patients. Both CT and MRI are useful to diagnose mycotic aneurysms. Treatment includes antibiotic therapy and surgical removal of the affected part of the aorta and revascularization of the lower extremities with grafts placed in uninfected tissue.

Syphilitic aortitis is a late manifestation of luetic infection that usually affects the proximal ascending aorta, particularly the aortic root, resulting in aortic dilation and aneurysm formation. Syphilitic aortitis occasionally may involve the aortic arch or the descending aorta. The aneurysms may be saccular or fusiform and are usually asymptomatic, but compression of and erosion into adjacent structures may result in symptoms; rupture also may occur.

The initial lesion is an obliterative endarteritis of the vasa vasorum, specially in the adventitia. This is an inflammatory response to the invasion of the adventitia by the spirochetes. Destruction of the aortic media occurs as the spirochetes spread into this layer, usually via the lymphatics accompanying the vasa vasorum. Destruction of collagen and elastic tissues leads to dilation of the aorta, scar formation and calcification. These changes account for the characteristic radiographic appearance of linear calcification of the ascending aorta.

The disease typically presents as an incidental chest radiographic finding 15–30 years after initial infection. Symptoms may result from aortic regurgitation, narrowing of coronary ostia due to syphilitic aortitis, compression of adjacent structures (e.g. esophagus), or rupture. Diagnosis is established by a positive serologic test, i.e. rapid plasma reagin (RPR) or fluorescent treponemal antibody. Treatment includes penicillin and surgical excision and repair.

Chapter 48

Cardiac Manifestations of Systemic Disease

Table 48.1: Cardiac manifestations of systemic disease

Systemic disorder	Common cardiac manifestations
Diabetes mellitus	CAD, atypical angina, dilated CMP (cardiomyopathy) and systolic or diastolic CHF
Protein-calorie malnutrition	Dilated CMP and CHF
Thiamine deficiency (beriberi)	High-output failure and dilated CMP
Hyperhomocysteinemia	Premature atherosclerosis
Obesity	CMP and systolic or diastolic CHF
Hyperthyroidism	Palpitations, SVT, atrial fibrillation and systolic hypertension
Hypothyroidism	Hypotension, bradycardia, dilated CMP, CHF, pericardial effusion and diastolic hypertension
Malignant carcinoid	Tricuspid and pulmonary valve disease and right heart failure
Pheochromocytoma	Paroxysmal hypertension, palpitations and CHF
Acromegaly	Systolic or diastolic heart failure and hypertension
Rheumatoid arthritis	Pericarditis, pericardial effusions, coronary arteritis, myocarditis and valvulitis
Seronegative arthropathies	Aortitis, aortic and mitral insufficiency and conduction abnormalities
Systemic lupus erythematosus	Pericarditis, Libman-Sacks endocarditis, myocarditis, arterial and venous thrombosis

Contd...

Contd...

Systemic disorder	Common cardiac manifestations
HIV	Myocarditis, dilated CMP and pericardial effusion
Amyloidosis	CHF, restrictive CMP and pericardial effusion
Sarcoidosis	CHF, dilated or restrictive CMP, ventricular arrhythmias and heart block
Hemochromatosis	CHF, arrhythmias, heart block and dilated CMP
Marfan syndrome	Aortic aneurysm and dissection, aortic insufficiency and mitral valve prolapse
Ehlers-Danlos syndrome	Aortic and coronary aneurysms, mitral and tricuspid valve prolapse
Addison's disease	Hypotension

In hyperthyroidism, a systolic pleuropericardial friction rub (Means-Lerman scratch) may be heard at the left second intercostal space during expiration and is thought to result from the hyperdynamic cardiac motion.

Chapter 49

Neoplastic Diseases of the Heart

Primary Tumors

- Primary tumors of the heart are rare.
- 75% are benign.
- Majority of these tumors are myxomas.
- Malignant tumors, almost all of which are sarcomas, account for 25% of primary cardiac tumors.

Clinical Presentation

- Cardiac tumors may present as chest pain, syncope, heart failure, murmurs, arrhythmias, conduction disturbances and pericardial effusion with or without tamponade.
- Additionally, embolic phenomena and constitutional symptoms may occur.

Myxoma

- Most common type of primary cardiac tumor in all age groups.
- They occur at all ages, most commonly in the third through sixth decades.
- With a female predilection, approximately 90% of myxomas are sporadic.

The Familial Variety

- Carney complex—(1) myxomas (2) lentigines and (3) endocrine overactivity (Cushing's syndrome, testicular tumors and/or pituitary adenomas with gigantism or acromegaly).
- NAME syndrome—Nevi, atrial myxoma, myxoid neurofibroma and ephelides.
- LAMB syndrome—Lentigines, atrial myxoma and blue nevi.
- Most are solitary.

- These are located in the atria particularly the left atrium, Where they usually arise from the interatrial septum in the vicinity of the fossa ovalis.
- Familial may be ventricular in location.
- Myxomas commonly present with obstructive signs and symptoms.
- The most common clinical presentation mimics that of mitral valve disease—Either stenosis owing to tumor prolapse into the mitral orifice or regurgitation resulting from tumor-induced valvular trauma.
- The symptoms and signs of myxoma may be sudden in onset or positional in nature.
- A characteristic low-pitched sound, a "tumor plop," may be appreciated on auscultation during early or mid-diastole.
- Myxomas also may present with peripheral or pulmonary emboli or with constitutional signs and symptoms, including fever, weight loss, cachexia, malaise, arthralgias, rash, digital clubbing, Raynaud's phenomenon, hypergammaglobulinemia, anemia, polycythemia, leukocytosis, elevated erythrocyte sedimentation rate, thrombocytopenia and thrombocytosis.
- Two-dimensional transthoracic or transesophageal echocardiography is useful in the diagnosis of cardiac myxoma.

Treatment

Surgical excision is indicated regardless of tumor size and is generally curative.

Other Benign Tumors

- Cardiac lipomas
- Rhabdomyomas
- Fibromas
- Hemangiomas
- Mesotheliomas
- Teratoma
- Sarcoma.

Tumors Metastatic to The Heart

- Tumors metastatic to the heart are much more common than primary tumors.
- The relative incidence is specially high in malignant melanoma and, to a somewhat lesser extent, leukemia and lymphoma.
- The most common primary originating sites of cardiac metastases are carcinoma of the breast and lung.

SECTION D

Investigations in Cardiovascular System (CVS)

50. The electrocardiogram
51. Noninvasive cardiac imaging
52. Stress tests
53. Cardiac catheterization

Chapter 50

The Electrocardiogram

An electrocardiogram (ECG or EKG) is a graphic recording of electric potentials generated by the heart.

ECG Waveforms and Intervals (Fig. 50.1)

- 'P' wave represents atrial depolarization.
- The QRS complex represents ventricular depolarization.
- ST-T-U complex (ST-segment, 'T' wave and 'U' wave) represents ventricular repolarization.
- The J point is the junction between the end of the QRS complex and the beginning of the ST-segment.

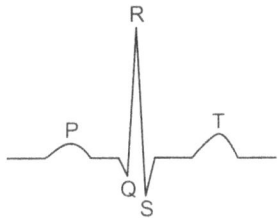

Fig. 50.1: Normal ECG

- ECG is recorded on graph paper that is divided into 1 mm² grid-like boxes.
- ECG paper speed is generally 25 mm/second.
- The smallest (1 mm) horizontal divisions correspond to 0.04 second (40 ms).
- With heavier lines at intervals of 0.20 second (200 ms).
- Vertically, the ECG graph measures the amplitude of a specific wave (1 mV =10 mm).
- There are four major ECG intervals: R-R, P-R, QRS and Q-T.
- The heart rate—1500/R-R interval in seconds.

- P-R interval—The time (normally 120–200 ms) between atrial and ventricular depolarization.
- QRS interval (normally 100–110 ms) reflects the duration of ventricular depolarization.
- The Q-T interval includes both ventricular depolarization and repolarization times and varies inversely with the heart rate.
- Corrected Q-T interval, QTc, can be calculated as QT/R-R and normally is 0.44 second.
- If the initial QRS deflection in a particular lead is negative, it is termed a 'Q' wave;
- The first positive deflection is termed as 'R' wave.
- A negative deflection after an 'R' wave is an 'S' wave.
- An entirely negative QRS complex is termed a QS wave.

ECG Leads

- The 12 conventional ECG
- Six limb (extremity) leads
- Six chest (precordial) leads
- The limb leads record potentials transmitted onto the frontal plane
- The chest leads record potentials transmitted onto the horizontal plane
  1. Lead V_1, fourth intercostal space, just to the right of the sternum.
  2. Lead V_2, fourth intercostal space, just to the left of the sternum.
  3. Lead V_3, midway between V_2 and V_4.
  4. Lead V_4, midclavicular line, fifth left intercostal space.
  5. Lead V_5, left anterior axillary line, same level as V_4.
  6. Lead V_6, left midaxillary line, same level as V_4 and V_5.
  7. Right precordial leads V_3R, V_4R, etc. detects evidence of acute right ventricular ischemia.

Electrical Axis

- It is determined from the frontal plane leads—I, II, III, aVR, aVL and aVF.
- It is quantified by using the hexaxial reference system (Fig. 50.2).
- The normal QRS axis shows a wide range of normality from −30° to +90°.
- Paired leads which are perpendicular to each other (lead I to aVF, lead II to aVL, lead III to aVR).
- Lead I and II show predominantly positive QRS complex—Normal axis.
- QRS complex predominantly positive in lead I and negative in lead III—Left axis.
- QRS complex predominantly positive in lead III and negative in lead I—Right axis.

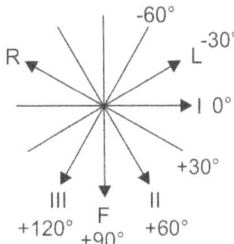

Fig. 50.2: Hexaxial reference system

- Left axis deviation is more negative than −30°.
- Right axis deviation is more positive than +90°.

Abnormalities

- Right atrial overload may lead to an increase in 'P' wave amplitude (2.5 mm).
- Left atrial overload produces a biphasic 'P' wave in V_1 with a broad negative component.
- Right ventricular hypertrophy—Tall 'R' wave in lead V_1, usually with right axis deviation.
- Left ventricular hypertrophy (LVH) by voltage criteria—SV_1 + (RV_5 or RV_6) >35 mm.
- Left ventricular "strain" pattern— ST depression + T inversion in lateral leads.

Acute Cor Pulmonale Due to Pulmonary Embolism

- Sinus tachycardia is the most common arrhythmia.
- Other tachyarrhythmias, such as atrial fibrillation or flutter, may occur.
- Right axis deviation.
- $S_1Q_3T_3$ pattern (prominence of the 'S' wave in lead I and the 'Q' wave in lead III, with 'T' wave inversion in lead III).

Bundle Branch Blocks

Wolff-Parkinson-White (WPW) syndrome

The diagnostic triad consists of
- Wide QRS complex associated
- Short P-R interval
- Slurring of the initial part of the QRS (delta wave).

Myocardial Ischemia and Infarction

- Acute infarction—ST elevations.
- Hyperacute infarction—Tall peaked 'T' waves.

- Acute subendocardial ischemia—ST-segment depression.
- Acute transmural anterior wall infarction is reflected by ST elevations in one or more of the precordial leads (V_1–V_6) and leads I and aVL.
- Inferior wall ischemia produces changes in leads II, III and aVF.
- True posterior wall MI – R/S ratio more than 1 in V_1, upright T and ST depressions in leads V_1 – V_3.
- Right ventricular ischemia usually produces ST elevations in right-sided chest leads—V_3R and V_4R.
- ST elevations are the earliest sign of acute infarction, followed by evolving 'T' wave inversions and often by 'Q' waves.
- Reversible transmural ischemia due to coronary vasospasm—Prinzmetal's variant angina may cause transient ST-segment elevations without development of 'Q' waves.
- Pseudonormalization—Patients whose baseline ECG already shows abnormal 'T' wave inversions may develop 'T' wave normalization during episodes of acute transmural ischemia.
- Wellens 'T' waves—Prominent 'T' wave inversions in the precordial leads in severe anterior wall ischemia.
- 'Q' wave infarction—Transmural infarction.
- Non-'Q' wave—Subendocardial (nontransmural) infarction.

Brugada Pattern (Fig. 50.3)

- Right bundle branch block-like pattern
- ST elevations in right precordial leads.

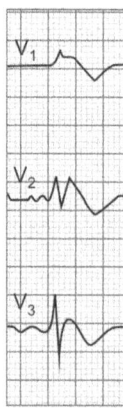

Fig. 50.3: Brugada pattern in ECG

Hyperkalemia (Fig. 50.4)

- Tall, narrow peaked (tenting) of the 'T' waves.
- Widening of the QRS interval.
- Severe hyperkalemia eventually causes cardiac arrest with a 'sine wave' pattern followed by asystole.

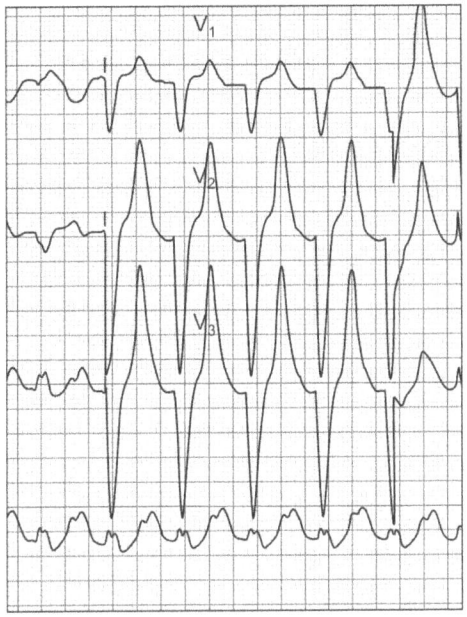

Fig. 50.4: ECG in hyperkalemia

Hypokalemia (Fig. 50.5)

- Prominent 'U' waves.
- Prolongation of the Q-T interval.

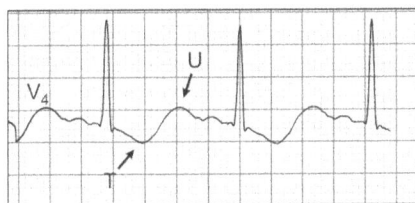

Fig. 50.5: ECG in hypokalemia

- **Systemic hypothermia**—Convex elevation of the J point (Osborn wave) (Fig. 50.6).
- Hypocalcemia—Prolongs the Q-T interval

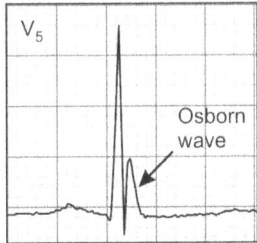

Fig. 50.6: Osborn wave in ECG

- Hypercalcemia—Shortens the Q-T interval
- Digitalis effect—Digitalis shorten the Q-T interval with "scooping" of ST–T wave complex.

Electrical Alternans (Fig. 50.7)

- A beat-to-beat alternation in one or more components of the ECG signal.
- Seen in pericardial effusion, usually with cardiac tamponade.

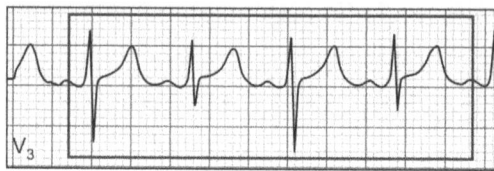

Fig. 50.7: ECG in electrical alternans

Chapter 51

Noninvasive Cardiac Imaging

Echocardiography

- Two-dimensional (2D) echocardiography is able to visualize the heart directly in real time using ultrasound, providing instantaneous assessment of the myocardium, cardiac chambers, valves, pericardium and great vessels.
- Doppler echocardiography measures the velocity of moving red blood cells and has become a noninvasive alternative to cardiac catheterization for assessment of hemodynamics.
- Transesophageal echocardiography (TEE) provides a unique window for high-resolution imaging of posterior structures of the heart, particularly the left atrium, mitral valve and aorta.

2D Echocardiography

- It is the "gold standard" for imaging valve morphology and motion.
- The imaging modality of choice for the detection of pericardial effusion.
- Intracardiac masses can be visualized on 2D echocardiography.
- It can provide extremely useful information on diseases of the aorta.

Doppler Echocardiography

- Doppler can be used to determine the pressure gradient across the valve.
- Valvular regurgitation is diagnosed by Doppler echocardiography when there is abnormal retrograde flow across the valve. Color-flow imaging is the Doppler method used.
- Intracardiac pressures can be calculated.
- Stroke volume and cardiac output can be reliably measured.
- Noninvasive evaluation of ventricular diastolic filling.

2D and Doppler echocardiography have been useful in the evaluation of patients with congenital heart disease.

Ejection fraction (EF)
- Represents the volume of blood pumped out of the left ventricle with each cardiac cycle.
- EF = Stroke volume/end diastolic volume × 100.
- Normal EF= 55–75%.

Stress Echocardiography
- 2D and Doppler echocardiography are usually performed with the patient in the resting state. Further information can be obtained by reimaging during either exercise or pharmacologic stress.
- The primary indications for stress echocardiography are to confirm the suspicion of ischemic heart disease and determine the extent of ischemia.
- Dobutamine echocardiography has also been used to assess myocardial viability in patients with poor systolic function.

Transesophageal Echocardiography
- Diseases of the aorta, such as aortic dissection, can be readily diagnosed by TEE.
- Defining the source of embolism is a common indication for TEE.
- The presence of vegetations for the diagnosis of infective endocarditis can be assessed by TEE.

Radionuclide Imaging
- This is uses of radioactive tracers to provide assessment of myocardial perfusion and metabolism, along with ventricular function.
- This is applied primarily to the evaluation of patients with ischemic heart disease.
- The two most commonly used technologies are single-photon emission computed tomography (SPECT) and positron emission tomography (PET).
- Assessment of myocardial perfusion and coronary artery disease—The most commonly used SPECT perfusion tracers are thallium-201 and technetium-99 labeled isonitriles.
- Assessment of myocardial metabolism and viability by PET scans.
- Assessment of ventricular function.

MRI/CT Imaging
- Cardiac MRI and CT scan can delineate cardiac structure and function with high resolution.

- They are useful in the examination of cardiac masses, the pericardium, the great vessels and ventricular function and perfusion.
- Gadolinium enhancement during cardiac MRI adds information on myocardial perfusion.
- Detection of coronary calcification by CT as well as direct visualization of coronary arteries by CT angiography (CTA) may be useful in selected patients with suspected coronary artery disease (CAD).

Chapter 52

Stress Tests

Definition

- Exercise testing is a cardiovascular stress test that uses treadmill bicycle exercise with electrocardiography (ECG) and blood pressure monitoring.
- Pharmacologic stress testing is a diagnostic procedure in which cardiovascular stress induced by pharmacologic agents like dobutamine
- Pharmacologic stress testing is used patients with decreased functional capacity or in patients who cannot exercise.
- Pharmacologic stress testing is used in combination with imaging modalities such as radionuclide imaging and echocardiography.
- Treadmill stress testing is indicated for diagnosis and prognosis of cardiovascular disease, specifically CAD.

Contraindications for Stress Testing

- Acute myocardial infarction within 2 days
- Unstable angina not previously stabilized by medical therapy
- Uncontrolled cardiac arrhythmias causing hemodynamic compromise
- Symptomatic severe aortic stenosis
- Symptomatic heart failure
- Acute pulmonary embolus or pulmonary infarction
- Acute myocarditis or pericarditis
- Acute aortic dissection.

Treadmill Protocol

- The standard Bruce protocol, includes 3 minute periods to allow achievement of a steady state before workload is increased.

- The modified Bruce protocol is most often used in older individuals or those whose exercise capacity is limited by cardiac disease.

Interpretation of Test Findings

- Interpretation should include exercise capacity and clinical, hemodynamic and ECG response.
- The occurrence of ischemic chest pain consistent with angina is important, particularly if it forces termination of the test.
- Positive stress test means an ST depression more than 1 mm.

Chapter 53

Cardiac Catheterization

Forssmann, Cournand and Richards are the pioneers of cardiac catheterization.

Cardiac Catheterization

Indications (Table 53.1)

Cardiac catheterization and coronary angiography are indicated to evaluate the extent and severity of cardiac disease in symptomatic patients and to determine if medical, surgical, or catheter-based interventions are warranted.

Table 53.1: Indication of cardiac catheterization

Coronary artery disease
High risk for adverse outcome based on noninvasive testing
Class III or IV angina on medical therapy
Unstable angina—High or intermediate risk
Chest-pain syndrome of unclear etiology
Acute myocardial infarction
Reperfusion with primary percutaneous coronary intervention
Persistent or recurrent ischemia
Severe pulmonary edema
Cardiogenic shock or hemodynamic instability
Mechanical complications—Mitral regurgitation and ventricular septal defect
Valvular heart disease
Suspected valve disease in symptomatic patients—Dyspnea, angina, heart failure and syncope
Asymptomatic patients with aortic regurgitation and cardiac enlargement or ejection fraction

Contd...

Contd...

Congestive heart failure
Congenital heart disease
Prior to surgical correction, when symptoms or noninvasive testing suggests coronary disease
Pericardial disease
Symptomatic patients with suspected cardiac tamponade or constrictive pericarditis
Cardiac transplantation

Contrast-induced nephropathy, defined as an increase in creatinine >0.5 mg/dl or 25% above baseline that occurs 48–72 hours after contrast administration, occurs in 2–7% of patients.

Vascular Access

- Cardiac catheterization procedures are performed using a percutaneous technique to enter the femoral artery and vein as the preferred access sites for left and right heart catheterization, respectively.
- A flexible sheath is inserted into the vessel over a guidewire, allowing diagnostic catheters to be introduced into the vessel and advanced toward the heart using fluoroscopic guidance.
- The brachial or radial artery may also be used as an arterial access site.

Right Heart Catheterization

- This procedure measures pressures in the right heart.
- It is done in patients with unexplained dyspnea, valvular heart disease, pericardial disease, right and/or left ventricular dysfunction, congenital heart disease and suspected intracardiac shunts.

Left Heart Catheterization

- This procedure measures pressures in the left heart.
- When aortic stenosis is present, there is a systolic pressure gradient between the left ventricle and the aorta.
- When mitral stenosis is present, there is a diastolic pressure gradient between the left atrial pressure and the left ventricle.

Table 53.2: Normal values for hemodynamic measurements

	Pressures (mmHg)
Right atrium	0–5
Right ventricle	

Contd...

Contd...

	Pressures (mmHg)
Peak systolic pressure	17–32
Pulmonary artery	
Peak systolic pressure	17–32
Pulmonary capillary wedge (mean)	4–12
Left atrium	4–12
Left ventricle	
Peak systolic pressure	90–140
Aorta	
Peak systolic	90–140
Resistances (dyn-s)/cm^5	
Systemic vascular resistance	900–1400
Pulmonary vascular resistance	40–120
Cardiac index [(L/min)/m^2]	2.8–4.2

Ventriculography and Aortography

- Ventriculography assesses left ventricular function, it may be performed during cardiac catheterization.
- Aortography visualizes abnormalities of the ascending aorta, including aneurysmal as well as dissection with compression of the true lumen.

Coronary Angiography (Fig. 53.1)

- It is used to define the coronary anatomy and determine the extent of coronary artery disease.
- Specially shaped coronary catheters are used to engage the left and right coronary ostia.
- Hand injection of radiopaque contrast agents create a coronary "luminogram" that is recorded on a radiographic images.
- Coronary angiography visualizes coronary artery stenoses as luminal narrowings.
- The degree of narrowing is referred to as the percent stenosis.
- A stenosis >50% is considered significant.
- Coronary calcification is also seen during angiography.
- Collateral blood vessels may be seen traversing from one vessel to the distal vasculature of a severely stenosed vessel.
- Thrombolysis in myocardial infarction (TIMI) flow grade provides a clue to the degree of severity of lesion.

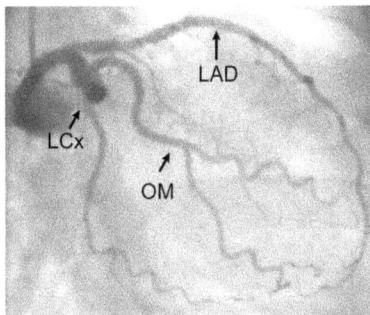 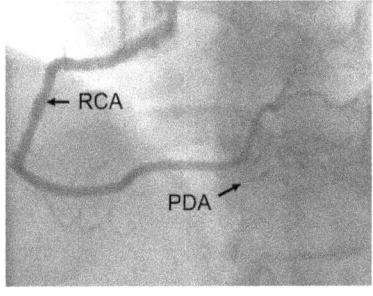

Fig. 53.1: Coronary angiogram

- Presence of TIMI grade 1 or 2 flow suggests that a significant coronary artery stenosis is present.

Fractional Flow Reserve

Measurement of the fractional flow reserve provides a functional assessment of the stenosis.

Index

Page numbers followed by *f* refer to figures and *t* refer to tables

A

Angina pectoris 5
Anginal equivalent 6
Angiography 228
Anomalous pulmonary venous connection 128
Aortic
  regurgitation 93
  stenosis 88
Atrial septal defect 109
AV node 178

B

Bendopnea 5
Blood pressure 30
Bradyarrhythmias 181
Broad complex tachycardia 179, 180
Bruit 151, 155, 180

C

Cardiac
  abnormalities 62, 129
  arrest
    cause 218
  cirrhosis 9, 135
  failure 132
  malposition 127
  tamponade 192
  transplantation 139
Cardiogenic shock 166
Cardiopulmonary resuscitation 164
Cardiovascular system 9, 11, 19, 65, 213
Cardioversion 82, 177
Catheterization with coronary angiography 167
Characteristics of anginal pain 6
Chest pain 79, 190
Closed mitral valvotomy 83
Clubbing 9
Coarctation of aorta 124
Collateral circulation 124
Complete transposition of the great vessels 130
Congenital
  aortic stenosis 88
  complete heart block 91
  heart diseases 109, 112, 127
Coronary arteriovenous fistula 61, 130
Coronary artery 16
Cyanosis 9, 101

D

Dextrocardia 127
Diabetes mellitus 136, 154, 158
Diagnosis of rheumatic fever 70
Dyspnea
  causes 3

E

Ebstein's anomaly 129
Echocardiography 76, 146, 156, 200, 202, 221
Ectopics 178
Ejection clicks 54
Electrical axis 216
Electrocardiogram (ECG)
  analysis of 172
  features 187
  in acute pulmonary embolism 50
  in arrhythmias 224
  in coronary artery disease 91
  in electrolyte imbalance 137
Embryology of the heart 14
Examination of neck veins 32

F

Fascicular blocks 187

G

Grading of
  dyspnea 3
  murmurs 56
    Austin-Flint 95
    continuous 59
    diastolic 57
    functional 62
    innocent 62
    Levine and Freeman's grading 56
    systolic 57
    to and fro 61

H

Heart
  block 181
  failure 132
    backward 133
    congestive 133
    forward 133
    left-sided 133
    right-sided 133
  murmurs 56
  sounds 191
    first 46
    fourth 52
    second 48
    third 51
Hemochromatosis 199*t*
Hemoptysis 8, 78
High-arched palate 107
High density lipoprotein (HDL) 157
Hypertension
  accelerated 166
  isolated 128
  malignant 10
  paradoxical 192
  systemic 148
  systolic 209
  transient 169
Hypertensive 148
  emergency 149
  states 37
Hypertrophic obstructive cardiomyopathy 8, 201
Hypertrophy 124, 139
  biventricular 139
  ventricular 124
Hypothermia 219
Hypothyroidism 175, 209

I

Indications for
  DC shock 177, 181
  permanent pacemakers 183
Infective endocarditis 10, 72
Inspection of precordium 37

J

Jones criteria 69
Jugular venous
  pressure 12, 32
  pulse 12, 34

K

Korotkoff sounds 27, 30, 31

L

Left
  atrial enlargement 41
  bundle branch block 186
  ventricular hypertrophy 124
Low density lipoprotein 157

M

Magnetic resonance imaging 200, 222
Management of
  DVT 140
  hypertensive crises 148
Midsystolic click 54
Mitral
  regurgitation 84
  stenosis 77
  valve prolapse syndrome 54
Myocardial infarction 85, 159
Myocarditis 195

N

Neoplastic diseases of the heart 211
New York Heart Association classification 3, 134*t*

Nonpharmacologic measures 137
Normal blood pressure 148

O

Obesity 4, 10, 40, 46, 140, 157
Open mitral valvotomy 83
Opening snap 80
Orthopnea 134
Orthostatic hypotension 7, 31

P

Palpation 12, 39
Parasternal impulse 41
Paroxysmal
   AV nodal reentrant tachycardia 173
   hypertension 209
   nocturnal dyspnea 4, 134
Patent ductus arteriosus 115
Percussion 12, 43
Percutaneous balloon valvuloplasty 83
Pericardial
   knock 44
   rubs 44
Pericardiocentesis 192
Pericarditis 189, 193
   acute 189
Pheochromocytoma 23, 209
Polymorphic VT 179
Potassium 158
Primary cardiomyopathy 198
Pulmonary
   angiography 142
   artery 37, 43, 81, 104, 146
   edema 79
   hypertension 78
   regurgitation 101
   stenosis 101
   thromboembolism 140
Pulsatile liver 135
Pulse
   character 11

   rate 11
   volume 11

Q

Q-wave 160

R

Radiofemoral delay 22
Radionuclide imaging 222
Restrictive cardiomyopathy 200
Rheumatic fever 67, 70, 97
Right 41
   atrial enlargement 106
   bundle branch block 185
   ventricular infarction 166
Risk factors for deep vein thrombosis 140

S

ST-segment 215, 217, 219
   depression 217
   elevation 219
Superior vena caval (SVC) obstruction 33
Syncope 7
Syndromes
   atrial septal defect (ASD) 109
   coronary 159
   Eisenmenger 121
   fetal alcohol 113
   Marfan's 85
   PDA 115
   sick sinus 181
   valve prolapse 54
   ventricular septal defect (VSD) 112

T

Tachyarrhythmias 172
Tetralogy of Fallot 117
Therapy
   antihypertensive 153
   pharmacologic 152
   quinidine 180
Thrills 41

Trepopnea 5
Tricuspid
   atresia 35
   regurgitation 35
   stenosis 35
Trifascicular block 188
Truncus arteriosus 130

U

Ultrasound 205, 221

V

Valve replacement 87
Valvular
   clicks 54
   heart disease 175
Vascular clicks 55
Ventricular septal defect 112

W

Wide pulse pressure 94

EU GSPR Authorised Reprsentative
Logos Europe, 9 rue Nicolas Poussin
1700, La Rochelle, France
Phone: +33 (0) 6 67 93 73 78
E-mail: contact@logoseurope.eu

www.ingramcontent.com/pod-product-compliance
Ingram Content Group UK Ltd.
Pitfield, Milton Keynes, MK11 3LW, UK
UKHW050455150426
5217IPUK00025B/1694